Flight OF FANCY?

Flights OF FANCY?

100 YEARS OF PARANORMAL EXPERIENCES

LYNN PICKNETT

WARD LOCK LIMITED·LONDON

DEDICATION

To

Uri Geller for changing the lives of millions

and

to Terry
simply with love

With thanks to:

Bob Rickard of the *Fortean Times* for his good humour, help and inspiration.

Sandi Bluestone for the word processing and Eric Taylor and Sheila Surgener for the typewriter that saved my life.

Joe Cooper for the Cottingley story and for being my partner in crime at conferences.

Professor Bob Morris (Koestler Chair of Parapsychology at Edinburgh University) for making me slightly more sympathetic towards his subject.

Peter Brookesmith for starting it all; Andrew Robinson for pointing me in the right direction; Sarah Litvinoff for believing that it could be done; and David, Helen and Anna at Ward Lock for seeing that it was.

First published in Great Britain in 1987
by Ward Lock Limited, 8 Clifford Street
London W1X 1RB, an Egmont Company

Text filmset in Sabon
by TJB Photosetting Ltd., South Witham, Lincolnshire.

Printed in Great Britain by
Butler & Tanner Ltd, Frome and London

British Library Cataloguing in Publication Data
Picknett, Lynn
Flights of fancy.
1. Psychical research
I. Title
133   BF1031

ISBN 0-7063-6526-7

▫ CONTENTS ▫

□ INTRODUCTION □

THERE IS A worldwide conspiracy in which, although we may not realize it, we all participate. Most of us are implicitly members at birth, but true initiation comes only when we reach the age of reason – when we acknowledge, no matter how reluctantly, that Peter Pan only flies with the aid of strings and pulleys, that miracles only happen to people in the bible (and perhaps not even then), that fairies, gnomes, angels and devils are folklore, and that Santa Claus is dead. On the day we are welcomed into the Great Conspiracy we receive a rule-book in which is inscribed just one rule: *avoid the impossible*. Then we are struck blind, deaf and dumb and patted on the head. From this position, we know where reality begins and ends. Dreams alone have the power to take us away from the bondage of this self-enforced freemasonry. We are grown-ups.

Frantically, we tell the world how to behave by drawing up a list of rules. The law of gravity, for example, encourages the belief that because most people do not suddenly float up to the ceiling, all levitation is humanly 'impossible'. But as we shall see, people do float and fly, extravagantly flouting our cherished rules. In retaliation we effectively ground them by declaring them, and their witnesses, liars and dupes.

Our conditioning as fully paid-up members of the Great Conspiracy means that we will do almost anything to obey the rule – *avoid the impossible*. Most of the time we don't even notice anomalous events, but if they are very intrusive we can always force them to fit civilization as we know it, rather like Cinderella's stepsisters and the glass slipper. If we can't blame a levitation or a ghost or spontaneous human combustion on something the Establishment (i.e. the High Command of the Conspiracy) will recognize, then we can always get ourselves certified insane before they do it for us. Like Cinderella's stepsisters who cut off their toes rather than admit the slipper did not fit, we will go to any lengths to fit the round peg of the paranormal into the square hole of the 'normal'. If we can't, then the tendency is to deny it ever existed. (Who wanted to marry the rotten old prince anyway?).

□

Consider the following examples of anomalous events and test your reactions to them:

□

In the 1980s a very down-to-earth British journalist was sitting outside a pavement-café in a backstreet of Paris. Suddenly the last car in the row parked across the street jumped of its own accord with such force that all the others in front shot forward a couple of feet. All the cars were empty and there was no one near.

In 1657, a young lad from Somerset was going about his business when he was abruptly lifted from the ground by an invisible power and levitated until his head touched the ceiling. He was then returned to the ground equally mysteriously. Henry Jones was afflicted in this way for a year; once he was thrown 27 m (30 yd) over a garden wall, but he was never hurt physically by these attacks. It was, of course, a grave offence to break the ground rules like this, and the neighbours were beginning to look askance, believing him to be bewitched. (If it happened today we wouldn't even allow ourselves that handy explanation to fall back on.) But fortunately, before the authorities asked him to help them with their enquiries, the tormentor, whoever or whatever it was, left him in peace. From then on Henry Jones kept his feet firmly on the ground like anyone else.

In 1904 in Falkirk, Scotland, neighbours found what they had to assume was the body of Mrs Thomas Cochrane, a well-connected widow, 'burned beyond recognition' lying on cushions and pillows that were not even singed. No one had heard her cry out and there was no fire in the grate nor any other source of fire or heat in the room. She had been destroyed by heat estimated in excess of 3000°F, yet it had failed to ignite the surroundings. This is typical of spontaneous human combustion (SHC).

In the mid-nineteenth century a Spiritualist medium, Daniel Dunglas Home, plunged his lily-white hands into the fire, lifting out red-hot coals in a borrowed handkerchief. Neither his hands nor the handkerchief showed the slightest signs of exposure to heat. He then conferred his incombustibility on the onlookers; when he handed them the live coals, they too suffered no damage and felt no heat.

At about the same time an Eastender, young Florrie Cook, regularly fell into a trance in her cabinet (a curtained-off recess) and shortly afterwards a woman in white emerged to walk among the sitters (those who attended the seances). She even perched flirtatiously on their laps and chatted inconsequentially to them. She claimed to be the physical materialization of a long-dead pirate's daughter, Katie King. Despite the fact that she looked *almost* exactly like her medium, many witnesses believed that she was indeed modern proof of the resurrection of the body – among them the eminent scientist William (later Sir William) Crookes.

To recognize the impossible you must suspend your disbelief which everyone is riddled with, as your reactions to the stories mentioned above no doubt reveal. Jumping cars? How many cognacs had the witness consumed? Or perhaps the driver had accidentally left something switched on, or something...anyway, cars do not behave in this way. At least one car did. Levitating boys? Well, it was in the wilds of Somerset way back in 1600-and-God-knows-when. Enough said.

Spontaneous human combustion (SHC) is very, very nasty as anyone who has read Dickens's *Bleak House* knows. But surely, we cry hopefully, that's just fiction? Unfortunately, Dickens based Krook's death on reports of real-life cases; it happened then and it happens now, despite coroners' elaborate attempts to explain away the horror: perhaps Mrs Cochrane was taken from her house and foully murdered by person or persons unknown, her body burnt and returned to her pillows where she was found? There is no evidence that this is what happened in this instance, nor in any of the dozens of other known cases of SHC. Uncomfortable though it is, the fact remains that people burst into flames apparently from within, while their clothes and surroundings escape undamaged. It could happen to you.

At the other extreme, human incombustibility as exhibited so flamboyantly by D.D. Home (and others, before and since) is absolutely impossible. We all know what happens if we play with fire. But then we have never tried it in the company of Mr Home.

And as for Florrie Cook and Katie King, the whole thing is a fraud and an insult to our intelligence. Miss Cook was clearly a confidence trickster (and very likely no better than she should be); moreover she is said to have confessed. QED.

Our first list of representative mysteries and miracles have been explained away, or at least enough doubt has been sown to make further investigation appear to be a forlorn exercise. Perhaps it's easier to relinquish our freedom and give ourselves back to the warmth and comradeship of The Conspiracy...?

Be absolutely clear on this point: making friends with the impossible is not for the faint-hearted or, and this may seem a paradoxical statement, for the gullible. After all, only the easily-swayed will disbelieve the testimony, of not only generation after generation, but even the evidence of their own eyes. As for the faint-hearted, the High Command, be they priests, scientists, or today's priest-scientists, have been known to take dissidents to one side with painful effect. Ordeal unto death by crucifixion, the rack, the stake, and trial by the media have been the fate of those who describe the real world as they have actually experienced it, rather than the world that operates according to the rules they know. Become a friend of the impossible and you automatically figure on someone's hit list. You have been warned.

Even if you are finally proved innocent of fraud and the phenomenon you have witnessed is accepted (very possibly disguised as a newly-discovered 'natural law') by the scientific brotherhood, don't expect them to apologize for their former scepticism. The frontiers of the 'possible' are always being redefined – that's 'progress' – but it's small comfort to those who were martyred for being ahead of their time.

The slow and painful tale of scientific discovery reads like a grim fairy story: Once upon a time, not so long ago, scientists sneered at the peasants who came running to them (this was in France actually, but it could have been anywhere). Great stones had hurtled out of the sky and crashed into the earth. Come, said the peasants to the scientists, and we will show you. But the scientists would not go to see for themselves, so the peasants brought some pieces of the stones to them. Pray do not bother us with your superstitions, said the scientists, they are merely rocks that have been struck by lightning. How can stones fall out of the sky when there are no stones in the sky? they scoffed. But meteorites kept falling just the same.

Early European explorers of the dark continent sent reports back to learned journals of their encounters with huge, hairy man-like monsters. What nonsense, said the professors in their gentlemen's clubs, it must be the effect of the heat (poor old Carruthers). But gorillas continued to exist nevertheless.

In our arrogance we believe we must give events permission to happen or creatures permission to exist. As the Book of Genesis says, 'In the beginning was the word...'. The existence of the Loch Ness monster was deemed a subject not even fit for debate until Sir Peter Scott gave the elusive creature a name: *Nessitera rhombopteryx*. Unfortunately, this mouthful was later discovered to be an anagram.

Rearrange the letters and you get: 'Monster hoax by Sir Peter S'...

With or without our puny acknowledgement, and outside of our control, the impossible has a field day. Unbolt the rivets of reason, remove the blindfold of dead knowledge, and see for yourself.

In 1986 millions of Wimbledon's tennis fans witnessed the short, sharp rebellion of a humble tennis ball against the tyranny of the Great Conspiracy. Live on television the rogue ball skimmed *through* the mesh of the net, exhibiting with true chutzpah which scientists and parapsychologists call 'matter through matter transference'. Even BBC's urbane commentator Dan Maskell was moved to muse that this was 'really quite remarkable', and viewers were treated to an action replay of what was, in effect, more a milestone in television and, indeed, human history than Armstrong's giant leap for mankind.

But the more outrageous the impossibility, the shorter our memories of it; play continued and the event did not even figure in the inevitable end-of-Wimbledon compilation of clips showing players falling over and umpires eating their sandwiches in the rain. Like many anomalous events it was spontaneous and over in a split second. Blink and you missed it, even given a brief action replay. Millions witnessed the event but how many remember it? It is part of our human condition, or rather human conditioning, that even viewers who remember it happening refuse to see its significance. A shrug and a yawn, a wave of apathy, actually masks our terror at the unleashing of the true, wild world we suspect hovers outside our five senses, like demons howling at the edge of the magic circle in which we live. If we allow ourselves to believe that our beloved, safe rules can be broken then perhaps they will, once and for all, fail us – with far more serious repercussions than a sudden rash of delinquent tennis balls. Chaos would rule.

Chaos, in fact, does rule, but only the brave dare acknowledge the fact. Making friends with the impossible means taking a firm stand; refusing to be brainwashed by the gullible materialists who have taken away our childhood. They are a motley crew but they tend to consist mainly of scientists who jealously guard their rule-making monopoly; conjurors, who would pay good money to learn the tricks of the impossible but if they can't then they become its implacable enemy; journalists, who see the impossible in terms of the great Sex Scandal – Peter Pan is really a girl (Shock! Horror!); and to a large extent, parapsychologists. This last category used to be called psychical researchers, but today it is mandatory to be an '-ology' to win the respect of the scientific Strong Arm Boys, and the grants at universities. As Bill Murray's parapsychologist says in *Ghostbusters*: 'Back off man, I'm a scientist...'

With a few notable exceptions, parapsychologists are 'moles' for the Great Conspiracy; they grovel to the Establishment and will never in a million years accept the impossible (unless they discover it for themselves). But more significantly, anomalous phenomena, by their very nature, will not obey the requirements laid down by Science. The paranormal (which is the impossible slowed down so we can perceive it) tends to behave like a particularly temperamental prima donna, who must be flattered and coaxed into giving her greatest performance – but she will only do it for her fans. Too often, parapsychologists turn the star into a ruined Judy Garland trying to croak her way over that rainbow while the audience throws bread rolls at her. Or, with scientific fervour they seek to strip, weigh and measure her – and what self-respecting star would allow that? As one friend of the impossible remarked, 'All this experimentation is like trying to make two strangers fall in love in a laboratory.'

To believe that anything can, and probably will, happen is to be free. And because the nature of the phenomena is whimsical we, too, as its friends, can be blissfully inconsistent in our favouritism: we may applaud D.D. Home and despise Florence Cook, look askance at fairies and ponder deeply about spontaneous human combustion, fire extinguisher to hand. Proof and disproof is from Alice-land anyway, whatever the men in white coats say. The paranormal puts on the motley, not rubber gloves.

If you make friends with the impossible it will make friends with you. The Cosmic Joker may have a wicked sense of humour, but he gets lonely laughing at his own jokes. We have stood in the corner too long – let's go out and play.

1

□ FLIGHTS OF FANCY? □

THERE IS, OF COURSE, A SOUND reason for ignoring the impossible in this life; on the whole our experience teaches that it is not advisable to handle live coals and that stepping out of a third-storey window with a view to floating in through the next one is a project with a limited future. Yet there have been those who are apparently incombustible, (just as victims of spontaneous human combustion are only too combustible) and others who – sometimes to their own embarrassment – defy the law of gravity and fly or float about in open defiance of the law said to have been formulated by the observation of an apple falling to the ground. It is remarkable that Sir Isaac Newton should have won such acclaim for noting such a common event, and that Daniel Dunglas Home, who did so much to prove that gravity is not binding, is largely forgotten.

Born in Scotland in 1833 and brought up by an aunt in America, D.D. Home (pronounced 'Hume') was a sickly, pampered child. He was believed to have strange powers, from an early age, which proved to be the case in spectacular fashion. When he was 13 he saw a vision of his friend Edwin, who was away from the neighbourhood at the time. The vision made three symbolic gestures in the air with its hands, then vanished. Home took this to mean that his friend had been dead for three days. This was, tragically, true. When his mother back in Scotland died, he saw her apparition before the news of her death arrived.

Thereafter, Home believed himself to be continually surrounded by the spirits of the dead, whose ministrations enabled him to produce astonishing phenomena and become, arguably, the greatest medium of all time. It never occurred to him to believe that the powers that helped him may have had a darker side, but when the house started to resound with mysterious rappings and crashings Home's aunt and uncle certainly thought him possessed by devils and threw him out.

Home's powers blossomed in an age hysterical with hauntings and resounding with the violent phenomena widely associated with poltergeists ('noisy spirits'). The birth of the Spiritualist movement, which was rapidly elevated into a religion, began with Kate and Margaret Fox in March 1848, in the hamlet of Hydesville, New York. The year before, their log cabin had been occupied by the Mitchell Weekman family, who had moved out when they discovered it to harbour an unwelcome guest. Rapping sounds issued from walls, doors and ceilings and their eight-year-old daughter screamed when a cold, disembodied hand touched her.

Twelve-year-old Kate Fox and her sister Margaret, aged fifteen, proved more than a match for the intrusive presence. They discovered that the raps could be made to answer questions (three knocks for yes, two for no and so on), through which they elicited the story of the unhappy ghost who plied them with its strange phenomena. It claimed to be a murder victim whose body was buried on their land and whose spirit was 'earthbound'. But the important aspect of this curious case was not the wretched ghost's tale, but the instant fame it brought the Fox sisters. Because they knew how to control the phenomena, and could reproduce them at will, they were seen to be the *mediums* through which the dead in the spirit world chose to contact the living. Suddenly Spiritualism and mediums were the rage, even surviving the confessions and retractions that beleaguer the world of the paranormal. It was into this welcoming atmosphere that Home was launched.

He rapidly made a name for himself as a

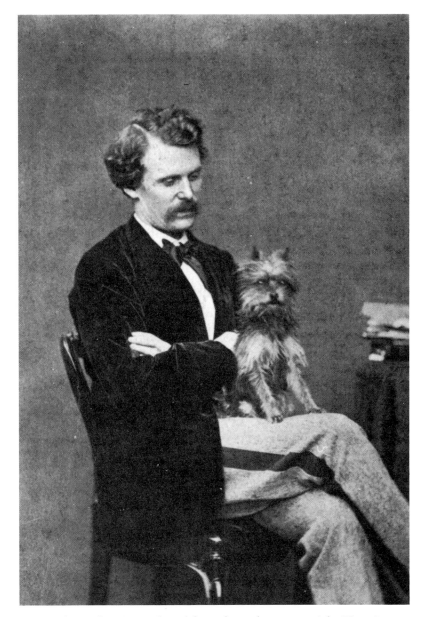

Daniel Dunglas Home, the celebrated – and controversial – Victorian medium, whose incredible feats are still hotly debated over 100 years after his death. His 'specialities' included levitation, incombustibility, bodily elongation, and the materialization of disembodied spirit limbs. Like Uri Geller, Home could also temporarily confer some of these strange powers on others; after handling live coals himself he would pass them to believers and sceptics alike, who also would suffer no ill effects then or later. Throughout his very public career he was never caught cheating nor seriously accused of it.

particularly talented Spiritualist who induced the usual repertoire of seance room phenomena with unusual flair: rappings apparently emanating from inside the very fabric of the furniture, floating lights, and irritable tables that lurched and tilted in answer to the sitters' questions. Victorian evenings could be very long indeed, and all the elements that made up a seance could result in a night to remember: semi-darkness, breathless expectation of some ghostly happening, and the heady delights of holding hands in the gloom. Fake mediums – there were estimated to be 1500 in the USA at the time – *always* ensured a good night's entertainment. When the genuine psychics were on top form they, too, could banish boredom in no uncertain manner. The competition was formidable, but one night in August 1852 at the home of a Mr Ward Cheney, who was a Connecticut businessman, Home's career literally took off.

THE IRRESISTIBLE RISE OF MR HOME

A local journalist, F. L. Burr, was present on this memorable occasion. His assignment was to find something incriminating against Spiritualism in general and Home in particular. However, instead of penning the ultimate exposé, Burr wrote:

> Suddenly, without any expectation on the part of the company, Home was taken up into the air. I had hold of his hand at the time and I felt his feet – they were lifted a foot from the floor. He palpitated from head to foot with the contending emotions of joy and fear which choked his utterances. Again and again he was taken from the floor, and the third time he was carried to the ceiling of the apartment, with which his hands and feet came into gentle contact.

Newton's apple had just gone up.

The act of flouting the law of gravity is known as levitation, and is most frequently associated with the stage magician's act in which a scantily-clad assistant (almost always female) appears to lie balanced on the points of swords. The swords are removed and *Voilà*! she lies in mid-air, rigid as if in a cataleptic trance, while hoops are passed over and under her to indicate the apparent lack of support. Sometimes, magic passes are made and she rises into the air (perhaps a trifle jerkily depending on the magician's skill). The act is a perennial favourite because levitation is regarded as impossible and hence, it is considered to be a very skilful trick.

But Home was not alone; throughout recorded history there have been incidents that prove levitation to be possible, rare perhaps, but nevertheless well-attested and, to some, an uncomfortable heresy.

A WING AND A PRAYER

At least two saints have experienced the ground being taken from under their feet by unseen agencies. St Teresa of Avila, an eminently sensible sixteenth-century Abbess and born organizer, whose feet should have been firmly on the ground, was also a mystic given to visions, trances and levitations that were often embarrassingly public. In her *Life* she wrote:

> It seemed to me, when I tried to make some resistance, as if a great force beneath my feet lifted me up...I confess that it threw me into great fear, very great indeed at first; for in seeing one's body thus lifted up from the earth, though the spirit draws it upwards after itself (and that with great sweetness, if unresisted) the senses are not lost; at least I was so much myself as to be able to see that I was being lifted up. After the rapture was over, I have to say my body seemed frequently to be buoyant, as if all weight had departed from it, so much so that now and then I scarce knew my feet touched the ground.

Sometimes this happened in church and the other nuns obligingly held her down to let the service continue in peace.

Just over twenty years after her death in 1582 a boy, Joseph, was born in Apulia, Italy whose single-minded devotion to a life of prayer naturally led him to the monastic life. One Sunday, the familiar drama of the Mass was being enacted when Joseph rose into the air and flew onto the High Altar – adding severe burns from the great phalanx of candles to the shame of showing off, in no uncertain manner.

A strange, withdrawn young man, a 'holy fool', in his utter simplicity he was not intellectually inclined like St Teresa, and left no personal record of his feelings about levitating. It is known that he, somewhat apologetically, referred to such incidents as 'my giddinesses' and that they happened frequently for they were a direct result of his excitement – and he was often excited. His fellow monks exhibited the usual reaction reserved for those who flaunt their 'impossible' powers – they shut him away for the rest of his life. But in the end it had to be admitted that he was a good monk, a better man, and that he actually did levitate. After his death he became St Joseph of Copertino, probably because several cardinals and Pope Urban VIII had personally witnessed his 'giddinesses'. (Neither he nor St Teresa is patron saint of those who levitate, but then the Roman Catholic Church today is a great believer in miracles, as long as they happened a long time ago.)

A life of prayer and meditation seems to clear one's personal flight path most efficiently. The French explorer Madame Alexandra David-Neel spent fourteen years in the mountains of Tibet, discovering for herself the truth about the legendary abilities of monks who fasted and prayed their lives away in those remote fastnesses. In her *Mystère et Magique en Tibet* (1931) she recalls meeting two men on a pilgrimage. One was naked, covered only in a cocoon of heavy chains. According to his companion only the chains held him down; without them he would float away, for his

spiritual life had made him virtually weightless.

On another occasion she saw a man covering enormous distances with huge, bounding leaps, impossibly long for most people. It was as if each step were less of a jump, more of a mini-levitation. A similar phenomenon was attributed to the legendary ballet dancer Nijinsky, whose high leaps were incredible enough, but it was the 'falling leaf' slowness of his return to the ground that was truly remarkable. Known as the 'slow vault', this controlled reluctance to come down to earth is said to be a secret skill handed down from generation to generation of peasants in remote rural areas of Europe and was practised in Russia, the dancer's homeland.

Today practitioners of transcendental meditation claim their discipline can enable them to levitate – one can, apparently, learn to fly just like the children in *Peter Pan* but more sedately, just a few inches off the ground.

In mid-nineteenth century USA there was only one who levitated without the aid of mirrors, machinery or even a safety net – the one and only D.D. Home, who described his phenomenal rise to fame thus:

> I feel no hands supporting me, and since the first time, I have felt no fear; though, should I have fallen from the ceiling of some rooms in which I have been raised, I could not have escaped serious injury. I am generally lifted up perpendicularly; my arms frequently become rigid, and are drawn above my head, as if I were grasping the unseen power which slowly raises me from the floor.

It is worth noting that, throughout his career, Home's feats regularly took place in houses he had not previously visited, among people he had only just met. The opportunity for rigging up elaborate machinery or engaging the services of an accomplice were extremely limited – and there is no evidence whatsoever to show that he ever resorted to such tricks. Quite simply, this was one medium (among a motley crew) who had no need to cheat.

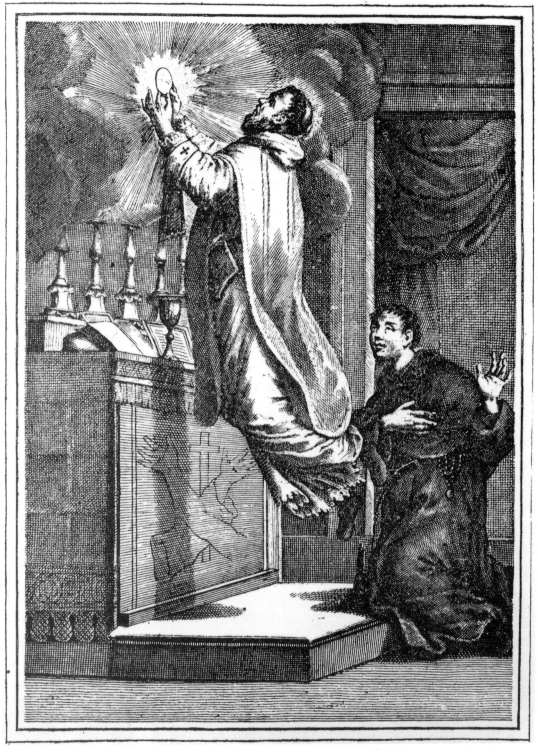

St Joseph of Copertino flies on to the High Altar during Mass. Like
St Teresa of Avila, this sixteenth-century monk was highly embarrassed by
the 'gift' of levitation, which seemed to confirm his sanctity.

A NIGHT TO REMEMBER

But it was in England, where he had been sent somewhat quaintly on doctor's orders, that he allegedly achieved his most controversial feat. In front of three irreproachable members of London's high society, Lord Adare, formerly a foreign correspondent for *The Daily Telegraph*, his cousin Captain Charles Wynne, and the Master of Lindsay, Home floated out of one window of a third-storey room some 24 m (80 ft) from the ground, and appeared at another moments later.

Although a true sceptic would simply dismiss all such 'impossibilities' as time-wasting rubbish, there is a peculiar breed of parascience parasite, who makes profit of one sort or another from 'exposing' the awesome, the wonderful, and those who 'merely' bend spoons. This curious leechlike creature is sometimes a scientist (for they make the rules that these psychics allegedly break), often a stage magician who feels himself slipping from the top of the bill, frequently a journalist and not infrequently a parapsychologist. What they have in common is an obsession with the paranormal and the desperate need to destroy it before it destroys their beautiful orderly world. Some of these missionaries for the rational (and the utterly boring) expose the same person several times, just to make their point and keep their own name in the headlines. Very rarely do they actually stop the impossible happening. The rabbit may no longer be in a particular hat, but it will pop up again somewhere else. Home, whose feats made him an obvious foe of sanity, had many enemies – and still does, a hundred years later.

John Sladek in his *The New Apocrypha* (1978) dissects and lampoons with the meticulous attention to detail one expects of the zealot; he, like all who truly believe their message, is persuasive (even though in his far-ranging demolition work he dismisses high-fibre diets as cranky). He set out to debunk Home's flight from reason that night so long ago by noting the discrepancies in the witnesses' statements about their experience:

> There was a ledge 4 inches wide below the windows (Adare); a ledge 1.5 inches wide (Lindsay); no foothold at all (Lindsay); balconies 7 feet apart (Adare); no balconies at all (Lindsay). The windows were 85 feet from the street (Lindsay); 70 feet (Lindsay); 80 feet (Home); on the third floor (Adare); on the first floor (Adare). It was dark (Adare); there was bright moonlight (Lindsay). Home was asleep in one room and the witnesses went into the next (Adare); Home left the witnesses in one room and went himself into the next (Adare).

They differed even on the basic fact of where the momentous incident took place: Lindsay said Victoria Street, Westminster and Adare said both Ashley Place, Westminster and 5 Buckingham Gate, Kensington in different statements. But to Sladek and others who seek to discredit Home (and to give them their due they would probably do the same even if he were able to reply to their accusations), the most damning aspects of the incident were Captain Wynne's simple description of the evening: 'Home went out of one window and came in at another', and the promise Home extracted from these upright British gentlemen that they would stay seated and not attempt to look out of the window during his 'flight'. Investigation was forbidden.

The counsel for the prosecution rests his case, having convicted D.D. Home of the fraud nearly a hundred years after the medium's death. Yet during Home's spectacular career he was never seriously accused of fraud – and never caught cheating like so many mediums who, although genuinely gifted, fall back on trickery whenever the power leaves them. (Indeed, given the nature of the phenomenon he evoked, it is difficult to imagine how he could have cheated.)

But the counsel for the defence must have his turn: of Captain Wynne's singularly unsensational statement perhaps he should have remembered he was making notes for posterity, especially for Mr Sladek, but he had seen a great many astonishing things happen and his 'Home went out of one window and came in another' might well have struck him as perfectly plain shorthand (rather as one poltergeist victim noted in her diary 'Rappings again since 3.30 a.m. Pools of water. Lights went out'). Even if Wynne had written: 'MEDIUM'S MID-AIR SENSATION, eye-witness exclusive!!!' he would have won Home no more friends. Besides, to a chap from a good school, sensationalism was distinctly 'bad form'.

A TUBERCULAR TARZAN?

In 1980 Archie Jarman reported in *Alpha* magazine that he had tracked down the building where the incident is said to have happened, discovering an 'Ashley Place' near Westminster Cathedral that had been called Ashley House in Home's time. On the top floor was a large room that tallied in detail with the descriptions given by those who had been present. The only major discrepancy was that the room was merely 13.5 m (45 ft) above the ground, but still quite far enough when attempting to walk on air. Jarman did notice a ledge 13 cm (5 in) wide running round the building just underneath the balconies, but a tentative experiment swiftly proved this to be an unreliable foothold. Only a stuntman or a well-equipped steeplejack would consider undertaking such a challenge, even across a mere 2 m (7 ft) gap between the balconies, and Home was neither.

In fact, when not entranced by his 'spirits', Home was hardly robust due to a tubercular condition – the last person to go fumbling about with tightropes on a chilly, dark December night in London. Furthermore, the major question remains: why would he want to? What motive could he possibly have for faking a stunt like that when he had performed considerably more startling feats before hundreds of others, a large proportion of them initially sceptical?

By far the most distinguished and prolific sceptic is Dr Trevor Hall, who finds the paranormal, especially Spiritualism, irresistible. In 1965 his *New Light on Old Ghosts* set out to show, by logical deduction from contemporary reports, that Home was at best an hypnotist and at worst a conjuror, claiming paranormal powers to enhance his reputation – the same allegation made against Uri Geller by envious conjurors today.

In 1985 Hall's *The Enigma of Daniel Home* (subtitled: 'Medium or fraud? The mystery of Britain's most famous spiritualist unravelled.') went over the same ground. Nearly a quarter of the book is devoted to the Ashley House case; Home's vanity (not disputed), alleged homosexuality (a recurring slur) and unscrupulousness (unproven) are presented like a statement for the prosecution. Where the evidence is open to other interpretation it has been omitted. As Professor Stephen E. Braude said in the correspondence pages of the *Journal of the Society for Psychical Research* (January 1986): 'It is quite ridiculous to suppose that one can make a sound sceptical case against Home, and never examine (even cursorily) the wealth of good material supporting the genuineness of his phenomena...most of Home's phenomena were observed under conditions far superior to those cited by Hall.'

If you don't like it, ignore it. The world seems cosier that way.

One of the features that appear to distinguish the true psychic superstar from the charlatan and the illusionist is the curious observation that their abilities are contagious. Home could levitate other people – on one occasion he levitated a woman together with the chair on which she was sitting. Members of the audience do not rise into the air when the stage magician levitates his assistant, just as there are never any reports of broken watches mysteriously mending or cutlery becoming unusable in the homes of viewers watching the tricks of James 'the Amazing' Randi or David Berglas.

One of Home's greatest enemies was Prince Metternich, who watched the medium's every move while they were both guests of the Emperor Napoleon III in January 1863. As was Home's way, the seance took place in a flood of light from the elegant chandeliers; he actually preferred to work his wonders in daylight or with some powerful illumination. He invited the sitters to observe him carefully, in direct contrast to the fashion for holding seances with eyes half-closed, holding hands in the dark. On this occasion the tablecloth rose into the air while Home and the sitters stood well away from it. This was Metternich's chance; he dashed forward and scrabbled under the table, eager to find some cunning machinery that Home had planted. The Prince was more than a little alarmed to find himself surrounded by a volley of loud raps emitting from within the fabric of the table. And there was no machinery.

The French Emperor employed conjurors and spies to catch Home out in some skullduggery, but they all confessed themselves beaten. In Rome his powers were ascribed, not to invisible strings and hidden accomplices, but to the work of the Devil; Home was requested very firmly to leave the Eternal City, never to float about its portals again.

His admirers and supporters vastly outnumbered his detractors, however. They included most of the titled heads of Europe, and men of learning – even the British physicist William Crookes, who was later knighted for his services to science. This bold and rare scientist reasoned that if such phenomena as those associated with Home did indeed exist then it was the duty of science to investigate them. He was to admit, however, in an article in the *Quarterly Review* (1870): 'At first, like other men who thought little of the matter and saw little, I believed that the whole affair was a superstition, or at least an unexplained trick.'

PAVING THE PATHWAY TO HELL?

But the sceptics had every reason to believe that Crookes was on their side, for in July of that year he wrote: 'The increased employment of scientific methods will produce a race of observers who will drive the worthless residuum of Spiritualism hence into the unknown limbo of magic and necromancy.'

In fact, Crookes was already a Spiritualist. He had confided to his diary that his private sittings with a medium called Mrs Marshall had convinced him that his brother, 'who passed over the boundary when in a ship at sea more than three years ago' continued to exist in the spirit world, and could communicate through mediums. To be fair to Crookes, what he had actually said was that he hoped scientific method would eliminate 'the worthless residuum of Spiritualism', presumably in order to sift out the dross and leave the shining nuggets for all to admire.

He found Home's attitude unusual in a contemporary Spiritualist medium – there was no forbidden territory of the sacrosanct cabinet, no enveloping darkness, no ifs and buts. Home said to Crookes: 'Now, William, I want you to act as if I was a recognized conjuror, and was going to cheat you and play all the tricks I could...Don't consider my feelings. I shall not be offended.' Among Home's phenomena Crookes listed:

- Movement of heavy bodies with contact, but without physical pressure.
- Currents of air.
- Changes of temperature (recorded on thermometers).
- Percussive noises – sometimes raps, but sometimes faint scratchings, sometimes detonations.
- Alteration in the weight of objects.
- Movements of furniture with no contact.
- Levitation of furniture with no contact.
- Levitation of Home himself.
- Movements of articles at a distance.
- Tunes of musical instruments which nobody was playing.
- Luminescences.
- Materializations, of human forms and faces.
- Materializations of hands (luminous or visible in light).

- Automatic writing. (Pens taken up by an invisible agency that wrote messages.)
- Phantoms.
- Telepathy (or the producing of information to which Home did not have direct access).
- 'Apports', (The Spiritualist term for objects that appear from nowhere and apparently move through solid matter, such as walls or ceilings.)

(Crookes omits to mention Home's incombustibility.)

In all the reports of these bizarre happenings there is not one that describes any sense of terror, or evokes the 'creepiness' usually associated with seance rooms. Home's sittings were conducted in a spirit of relaxed expectation, of normal conversation and laughter – as we shall see, this kind of atmosphere can be very powerful in inducing paranormal phenomena, whether one believes in spirits or not.

Trevor Hall, however, finds: 'The oddly credulous flavour of Adare's account, and the multiplicity of the alleged phenomena...which he described as casually as if they were "everyday occurrences", can, I think, be regarded as significant.'

Anybody reporting what Adare had seen would sound credulous and to Home, at least, the phenomena were indeed 'everyday occurrences'. To holy men and shamans of many allegedly 'primitive cultures' the impossible is a way of life, only the perspective is different. As Edward Tylor, the Victorian anthropologist mused, it appears that 'the Red Indian medicine man, the Tartar necromancer and the Boston medium share the possession of a belief and knowledge of the highest truth and import which, nevertheless, the great intellectual movement of the last two centuries has simply thrown aside as worthless.' Since Tylor wrote in the mid-nineteenth century, the number of babies thrown out with the bathwater by fanatical debunkers amounts to genocide.

Enemies of the impossible also tend to lump together medicine men, necromancers, mediums (and metal-benders) as pedlars of pernicious nonsense. In the terminology of contumely, if 'ignorant savage' won't fit, then substitute 'unscrupulous charlatan'. The bigger the reputation of the miracle worker in question, the higher the price he or she must pay for fame and (in a very few cases) fortune. Home was a high-flyer in more ways than one, a prime target for the slings and arrows of outraged rationalists, and although not one of them has been able to show Home's phenomena to have been fraudulent, they perform their own illusion by pretending that they have. And as reputations are lined up against the wall to be shot, they might as well eliminate one of the ring-leaders – William Crookes.

As Sladek says, 'When an eminent scientist gets involved with the supernatural in any capacity, believers rejoice.' But this is taking a quote out of context, for it refers to his investigation of the mediumship of Florence Cook (of which more later). Perhaps the debunker thinks his hatchet-job on the Cook-Crookes research is retrospective death and damnation to all his earlier investigation into Spiritualism. (But if Crookes' study of Home was lies, that with Florence Cook was 'damned lies...')

It seemed perfectly reasonable to Crookes that if Spiritualist phenomena exist then it is the responsibility of science to investigate them.

Crookes was not much concerned with the psychology of the events, but concentrated his research along well-established experimental principles. As he said:

The spiritualist tells of bodies weighing 50 lb or 100 lb being lifted up into the air without the intervention of any known force; but the scientific chemist is accustomed to use a balance which will render sensible a weight so small that it would take ten thousand of them to weigh one grain; he is, therefore, justified in asking that a power, professing to be guided by intelligence, which will toss a heavy body up to the ceiling, shall also cause his delicately-poised balance to move under test conditions.

Much intrigued by the phenomena of Home's flying accordion, Crookes devised a copper cage, in which it was secured. Home was allowed to touch the apparatus only at the point furthest from the keyboard. Nevertheless it began to play a medley of popular tunes, and continued to do so for a short while even after Home had taken his hands away. The accordion and its cage is now in the possession of the Society for Psychical Research (SPR). Formed by a distinguished group of Cambridge scholars in 1882, originally to study telepathy between the living, the Society has latterly become obsessed with the 'scientization' of the paranormal, with the predictable result that it attracts more foes than friends of the impossible. Interestingly, however, Home is still a big enough name for serious criticism of him to provoke a flurry of protests in its *Journal*. A sensitive in every sense of the word, Home was fortunate to live before the advent of psi-stifling, white-coated parapsychology.

Home's stature as a medium continued to grow – literally. At a seance in 1867 Lord Adare noted: 'Standing there beside me, Home grew, I should say, at least six inches.' John Sladek and other debunkers would sniff at taking the word of a witness who had confused the details of Home's controversial 'flight' at Ashley House, Westminster, but fortunately there were many others who attested to the extraordinary sight of Home's body elongating, even with strong men holding on to his legs and trunk. It seemed as if his ribcage rippled as an implacable force drew him upwards.

PLAYING WITH FIRE

But for many, Home's most incredible ability was his incombustibility; when entranced, his hands 'soft and delicate like a woman's' would pluck out live coals from fires, and he could even lie with his face buried in white-hot cinders without any damage, then or later. Sometimes he wrapped the coals in handkerchiefs borrowed from others in the room, returning them unsinged. But most significantly he could pass on this bizarre ability temporarily to others. Crookes recorded that:

> Home removed from the grate a red-hot piece nearly as big as an orange, and putting it on his right hand, covered it with his left hand so as to almost completely enclose it, and then blew...until the lump of charcoal was nearly white-hot, and then drew my attention to the lambent flame which was flickering over the coal and licking round his fingers...

Adare, Lindsay and Wynne were again on hand when Home re-enacted the miraculous events of the New Testament Pentecost, when the Apostles had received the gift of the Holy Spirit. Tongues of flame shot from the medium's head, then Adare reported: '...we all distinctly heard, as it were, a bird flying round the room, whistling and chirping. There then came the sound of a great wind rushing through the room; we also felt the wind strongly.'

Brian Inglis has also pointed out the connection between Home's phenomenon and the bodily elongation of the saints, who were reported to be drawn upwards while their feet remained on the ground, as depicted in the paintings of El Greco.

This is not to imply that Home himself was a saint, although he maintained the belief that his psychic gifts were manifestations of the agency of beneficent spirits. Despite the Christian supposition that those who do good, or have amazing powers, must themselves live modest and saintly lives, the facts do not bear this out. At least one of today's top healers has manners that would disgrace a pig, and neither Home nor his modern counterpart, Uri Geller, is known for his modesty. It seems that psychic gifts, like a talent for doing impressions or playing the bagpipes, are no respecters of persons. Whatever triggers paranormal abilities in certain individuals may be connected with their beautiful souls, but this is unlikely.

Home was unsparing in his comments on other mediums of his day:

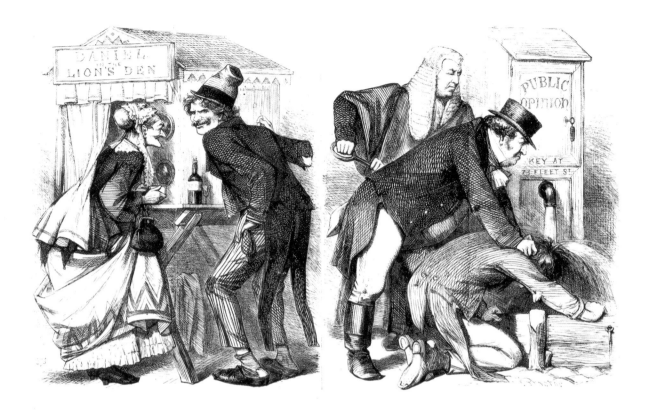

'Spirits and water', one of the vicious cartoons that appeared in 1868 when
D.D. Home was accused of extorting money from a rich old lady,
Mrs Jane Lyons. It was the lowest point in his career.

The wildest imaginings of the Catholic children, who beheld 'the Virgin washing her feet
in a brook', have been more than paralleled
among spiritualists. Some years ago our cause
rejoiced in a 'medium' of twelve years old,
who was assuredly a highly favoured boy.
Angels of the most select class guarded him.
The chief band was no less a personage than
the Virgin. Herself and coadjutors possessed,
it was declared, an insatiate appetite for
plum-pudding and dried fruits. I have myself
heard the uncle of the lad in question relate,
with the gravest conviction, how at their
seances spirit voices would suddenly speak
from out the darkness, telling the sitters, 'here
we are! The Virgin Mary's coming, get out the
sherry wine and the raisins.'

Perhaps Home had every reason to feel
complacent, but even he had his problems. For
a time, Mrs Jane Lyons, a rich widow, took him
up, settling the not inconsiderable sum of
£60,000 on him and making him her heir.
Although Home never normally accepted
money for seances he took this sum, on his
friends' advice, and almost immediately found
himself in the dock, accused of extorting the
money by alleging to Mrs Lyons that the spirits
wanted her to give him it. The judge, no friend
of Spiritualism, attacked the widow's testimony in no uncertain terms, declaring that
she had made '...misstatements on oath so per-
versely untrue that they have embarrassed the
court to a great degree, and quite discredited

the plaintiff's testimony.' However, he granted Mrs Lyons her money back, 'for as I hold Spiritualism to be a delusion, I must necessarily hold the plaintiff to be the victim of delusion.' Spiritualism lost the case, not Home. Nevertheless, it gave his enemies much needed ammunition and mud, once thrown, tends to stick.

SLUDGE, SLURS AND SLIME

In Britain Home was a powerful influence in the thinking of such luminaries as Lord Lytton, John Ruskin, Charles Dickens, and Elizabeth Barrett Browning. The husband of the latter, Robert, was to become his bitter enemy and lampooned him, and Spiritualism in general, unmercifully in his *Mr Sludge the Medium*, written in 1864. It seems that sheer jealousy was the motive behind this vindictive poem of Browning's; in 1855 Home had given a private sitting in the Brownings' house, during which a wreath of clematis rose into the air and finally came to rest on Elizabeth's head. Robert followed it around the room, and Home suggested that perhaps he wanted it to settle on his brow. One theory is that this petty incident, reminiscent of playground sniping, laid the foundation for Robert's festering hatred of the medium. It seems more likely that it was triggered simply by Elizabeth's open espousal of Spiritualism, and in particular, her championship of D.D. Home. To make matters worse in the Browning household, Elizabeth's poetic career was in the ascendant while Robert's was static.

At the time of the clematis-wreath incident, however, none of Robert's letters indicate that he considered Home to be a fraud, but with the passage of time he came to believe that he had himself detected Home in an act of trickery. Elizabeth never wavered in her belief in Home's powers, and significantly, *Mr Sludge* was published only after her death.

Among his distinguished supporters, however, Home could count his brother-in-law, a respected Russian scientist, Alexander von Boutlerow, who conducted his own investigations into the medium's paranormal powers some years before Crookes. Home's first, and much beloved, wife died young. Later, during a visit to the court of the Russian Tsar, he fell head over heels for Julie de Gloulemine. The attraction was mutual, and they married.

Boutlerow was intrigued by the possibility that his brother-in-law was a brilliant hypnotist, causing people to *think* they saw tables rising into the air, while the furniture actually remained, as experience predicts, firmly on the ground. One of Home's favourite parlour games was to get the sitters to command a heavy table *not* to move, then try and levitate it – lo and behold it stayed where it was (not surprisingly, say the sceptics). Then when they commanded it to rise – up it floated. Was the real table on the ground all the time and the levitating table all in the mind? (Peter O'Toole's mad Earl in *The Ruling Class*, believing himself to be Jesus, almost manages a similar feat, but the song and dance routine of Arthur Lowe's drunken butler brings the gathering to its senses.)

Boutlerow designed an ingenious weighing device for recording the difference, if any, between the table when at rest and when it took off. A table weighing 45.4 kg (100 lb) with its feet on the ground was shown to gain an enormous 68 kg (150 lb) when commanded like a dog to 'stay', but lost a phenomenal 32 kg (70 lb) when, with Home resting his fingertips on its top, it was instructed to rise. Can instruments be hypnotized?

WITH A LITTLE HELP...

Home was perhaps somewhat over-qualified to preside over that particular 'trick'. Anybody can do it, as the thousands could have told him who have played the levitation game (that was to become fashionable in British playgrounds and pubs). The layman's version involves people, not tables. What you do is this:

Choose the heaviest person in your group – the hardest part may turn out to be the tact required – but the heavier the person, the more impressive the result. Sit him (or her) in a chair. Four of you then proceed to prove it's impossible to budge him, let alone cause him to rise into the air, by hooking your index fingers in the crooks of his elbows and behind his knees. Like the table commanded to remain doggo, he sits on. Then you all pile your hands on his head, interleaving them, and say a magic word – 'Abracadabra' will do – this is not a test of originality. Immediately after this you repeat the process of trying to lift up your too, too solid friend with fingers alone. It works. Up he goes. All good, harmless fun that beats dominoes any day. But the joke is once it moves out of the realms of fun and into the laboratory it won't work. Worse, you'll all begin to wonder if it ever had worked – maybe it was 'just imagination' (whatever that is).

Home's version had the edge because it did work for a scientist, but even so the phenomenon was recorded in a drawing room, surrounded by believers who were having a good time. Nothing inhibits showpiece psychokinesis (PK, or mind over matter) more than a negative attitude. The impossible is least intrusive when one is 'down' or in a rut. (Recent research indicates that the most bizarre things tend to happen to people on holiday, when they're happy and routine is forgotten.)

One of the most successful psychokinesis groups of modern times – and naturally one of the most controversial – is SORRAT (the Society for Research on Rapport and Telekinesis) founded by the poet and mystic Dr John G. Neihardt in 1961 in Missouri, USA. For over twenty years, a group averaging fifteen sitters attended meetings, hoping to induce such things as table-tilting phenomena and 'spirit' rappings. Some, but not all, of the group were Spiritualists. Their patience was finally rewarded beyond their wildest dreams.

Dr Neihardt's home, the picturesquely named Skyrim Farm, soon resounded with paranormal rapping; tables tilted and even 'walked'; objects levitated and at least one regular sitter went into a trance. But it was the minilab, created by researcher William E. Cox,

that trapped the most astonishing phenomena, which were also recorded on film. Basically just an upturned aquarium sealed round the bottom, the minilab contained a number of objects, such as a pen and paper, leather rings, and packs of cards, for the 'entity' to play with. If the objects moved of their own accord, they triggered off a short burst of movie film, which although it had the disadvantage of working after the event (and the quality of the film was very poor), it often managed to capture scenes being enacted inside that simple fish tank that crashed the 'boggle threshold'. On one occasion, two leather rings rose into the air and linked themselves together, then one of them casually emerged through the solid glass wall of the minilab, falling on to the table underneath. This rare example of 'matter through matter transference' happened between the frames of the film. (Although it 'holds no corporate views' the Society for Psychical Research hates the Society for Research on Rapport and Telekinesis [SORRAT]. Its results are so 'impossible' that it almost seems like bad form to acknowledge its existence.)

Dr John Thomas Richards, SORRAT's historian, describes the atmosphere at an early meeting:

> We sang, talked, joked, and made a deliberate effort not to be somberly serious, since Dr Neihardt felt that a light approach to paranormal phenomena was more likely to put us into the best psychological frame of reference for positive results, as opposed to a mood which was reverential, awe-permeated, morbid or fearful. He believed that 'a happy, good feeling of unity was what the seance groups under Home and other fine mediums of the last century seemed to experience over and over again, and that did not mean that they became over-credulous. At the same time, they had outstanding success with levitation.'

But to many, Home's sudden surges of weightlessness were less impressive than his immunity to fire, which Adare and others had discovered to be temporarily contagious. When Home handled live coals without harm, so could others in the room. Saints, shamans and yogis have long been reported to possess protective power against extreme heat, which they could confer on others for as long as was needed. Stories abound of the famous Fijian firewalkers, whose immunity to heat extended to the ceremonial leaves attached to their ankles; even a slow walk over incandescent cinders failed to harm the men or their regalia. Their ordeal is preceded by secret rituals (which sceptics assume must include the lavish application of an undetectable protective substance, but is much more likely to be a trance-based shifting of consciousness to the magical level where men can work miracles).

Today, the 'coal stroll' is a natural extension of the consciousness-raising cults of California; anyone can walk on fire if his or her mental preparation is right. In England in 1985 people paid £50 each to learn how to walk over red-hot coals and emerge unscathed. The technique involved visualization (a potent method of bypassing ordinary consciousness and reaching the powerful subconscious), and chanting, which reinforces the images implanted in the imagination. The group thought of anything that was the opposite of burning red coal and went into the ordeal looking up at the stars, chanting 'Cool, wet grass, cool wet grass...' Very few of them were burnt and of those only a slight blistering occurred. All of them had been frightened before the walk. Afterwards there were hugs and kisses and laughter. Nothing makes life worth living more than achieving the impossible.

Home's continued fame rests on the sheer variety of phenomena he produced. Today a few individuals boast amazing, but comparatively limited, powers. American Jack Schwartz is virtually incombustible, and he can lie on a bed of sharp nails with a heavy man standing on him and remain unhurt and unpunctured. Uri Geller can mend, bend and – as with computers – break things and confer the abilities on others who watch or listen to him. Almost any group of people with enough

patience can, like SORRAT, get objects to behave as if they had minds of their own. But Home had an astonishing repertoire, as listed by Crookes (page 21).

John Sladek has this to say of these legendary abilities:

> A formidable list, and if Home had actually been able to perform almost anything on it, there would have been no room for scepticism. Alas, most of these phenomena were observed by Crookes alone, and no independent evidence exists of their having worked. When a man attests to incredible feats like levitation, we must be sure he isn't lying, that he hadn't been hallucinating, drugged or hypnotised [hypnotism was itself, until very recently, high on the sceptics' hit list], that he hasn't been fooled by conjuring tricks, and that he hasn't been coerced or persuaded into his testimony.

To paraphrase Mr Sladek, this is a formidable list of innuendo and slur, and if he had been able to prove anything on it, there would be no room for belief. As it is, there is absolutely no proof that Home was anything but genuine. The man Sladek clearly had in mind who attested to the 'incredible' feat of levitation was Lord Adare, who 'besides sharing his bed with Home, was otherwise under his influence.' Even if one accepts the homosexual jibe, surely the other 'influence' could well have been, quite simply, the natural admiration for Home's powers? Did the witnesses of St Teresa's levitations sleep with her or take drugs? (Or is their testimony automatically invalid because the phenomena happened a long time ago and to a saint? All saints are silly.)

The fact that, out of all his phenomena, Home's levitation was singled out for vilification by Sladek, and was a substantial part of Hall's allegations, says more about them than about Home. Loosening the bonds of gravity – or at least seeming to – is obviously much more disturbing to the Great Conspiracy than being impervious to fire or causing hands to

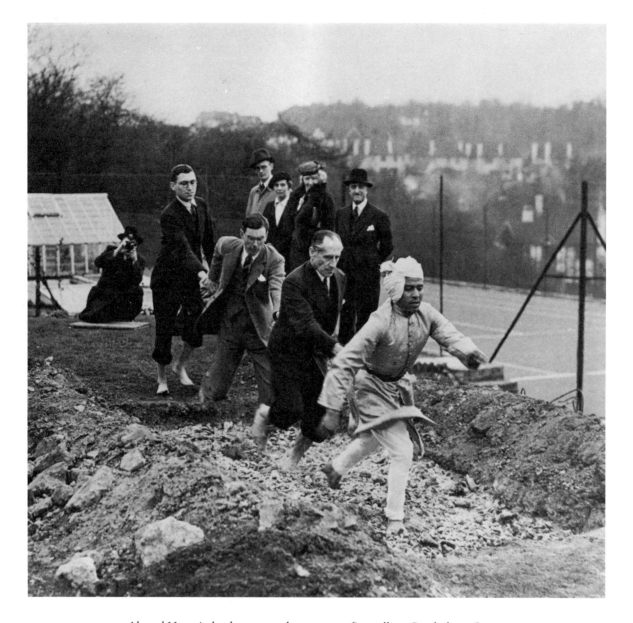

Ahmed Hussein leads a somewhat nervous firewalk at Carshalton, Surrey
in April 1937. The true 'coal stroll' can be undertaken by anyone in the
right state of mind; consciousness-raising techniques such as hypnosis
can induce sufficient 'mind over matter' to prevent burning of feet or
clothes. The trances of saints and mystics often made them temporarily
incombustible and a few rare Spiritualist mediums, such as D.D. Home,
also proved themselves a match for mere fire. One of Home's 'party
pieces' was to bury his face in the white-hot coals of a parlour fire or
appear to wash his hands in the glowing embers. The saints ascribed this
ability to the protection of God; Home believed his powers to come from
spirits of the dead. But the miracle was the same.

materialize out of thin air – although these, too, are dismissed as delusion or fraud. They would have Peter Pan grounded and Superman stopped. Man cannot fly; Icarus was proved wrong, we should know our place and keep our feet on the ground. *Know thyself* takes second place to *Know thy place*.

TO DREAM THE IMPOSSIBLE DREAM

Dreams of flying are very common, and are usually exciting and pleasurable rather than frightening – perhaps because, as the Freudians believe, they represent an orgasmic climax, or perhaps because they show us how it feels to be freed from the deadening pull of gravity, the encasement of the physical body.

A desire to fly seems to be strong in the human race. We seek the stars rather than explore the relatively unknown world of our oceans; under the influence of hallucinogenic drugs such as LSD we believe we *can* fly (and sometimes, tragically, prove we are wrong); our saints and mystics levitate or dissolve the bonds of the flesh in their ecstatic trances, which are themselves often a form of flying:

The Victorian vicar's daughter whose passionate genius gave us *Wuthering Heights* lived a strange double life. Emily Brontë's day was similar to those of many another shabby-genteel lady in the 1840s – supervizing the cooking and washing for the household, and often rolling up her own sleeves to help bake the bread. But at night, even after she had retired to scribble the darkly disturbing tale of Heathcliff and Cathy, another kind of experience overtook her, shaking her frail body and engulfing her whole being in a kind of spiritual flame. The gruff, shy girl who preferred the kitchen to the company-best parlour became a mystic just as the equally practical St Teresa had three centuries before. Emily Brontë flew – not as visibly as her saintly counterpart – but she was spiritually elevated to an intense rapture, the mystic's ecstasy.

She describes this bliss, and the pain of its

ending, in these verses, taken from 'Julian M. and A.G. Rochelle' (9 October 1845):

> But first a hush of peace, a soundless calm
>   descends;
> The struggle of distress and fierce impati-
>   ence ends;
> Mute music soothes my breast – unut-
>   tered harmony
> That I could never dream till earth was
>   lost to me.
>
> Then dawns the Invisible, the Unseen its
>   truth reveals;
> My outward sense is gone, my inward
>   essence feels –
> Its wings are almost free, its home, its
>   harbour found;
> Measuring the gulf it stoops and dares the
>   final bound!
>
> Oh, dreadful is the check – intense the
>   agony
> When the ear begins to hear and the eye
>   begins to see;
> When the pulse begins to throb, the brain
>   to think again,
> The soul to feel the flesh and the flesh to
>   feel the chain.

The psychical researcher calls such experience 'out-of-the-body-experiences' (OOBEs), although modern case histories are not restricted to the religious or mystical rapture. Physical shock or pain, anaesthetics or clinical death can free the spirit, or consciousness, from the bonds of the body. A delightful feeling of floating or soaring is the most common sensation of an OOBE, but in many cases it seems to let the person experiencing it impinge on the real world in tangible ways. A little girl, hovering in delirium between life and death slipped out of her body and sat invisibly in her doctor's car as it stopped at the traffic lights. He was somewhat surprised when his patient told him precisely what he'd been muttering under his

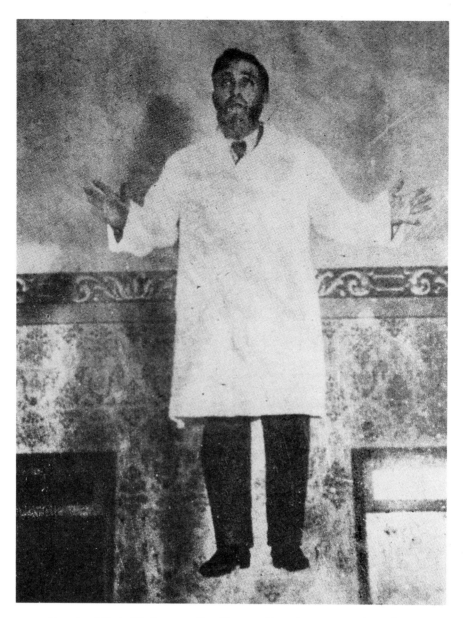

Carmine Mirabelli, the great Brazilian medium, hovers near the ceiling, without benefit of string, pulleys, or a safety net. There are some who believe that his extraordinary career matched that of D.D. Home; certainly the range and theatricality of his abilities were spectacular and had the added benefit of being captured by the camera. Sceptics believe levitation to be impossible – the product of mass hypnosis or collusion. Any theory is more comforting than the possibility that gravity is not binding.

breath en route to her bedside. Even more of an embarrassment was the free-floating young man whose seriously sick body was undergoing surgery; his consciousness took time out to wander the hospital and eavesdrop on some juicy gossip, which he duly repeated to the scandalmongers themselves after he came round from his operation...

Almost everyone who experiences an OOBE hates 'coming back'. They have been free; they have flown. Perhaps there is some truth in the ancient belief that a split-off part of our personality escapes during sleep, to pursue its own adventures that our integrated selves on waking recollect only fragmentarily, all jumbled up. 'We are such things as dreams are made on', Shakespeare said. Recent research has shown that OOBEs are not restricted to the mystic or the drug addict – they seem to be just below the surface waiting for some trigger to release them. (And the ultimate trigger is the death of the body: freedom at last?)

Perhaps those rare beings who find themselves levitating physically are subconsciously releasing the trigger and allowing an enormous surge of the energy used in OOBEs to take hold of their bodies and up they go, briefly. Hypnosis has proved the power of the mind over the body: horrifying skin conditions clear up, people whose traumatic experiences have made them blind or dumb can see and speak under its influence – so how much more powerful then is the whole spirit over the body? (This is careless talk as far as the sceptics are concerned, to speak of the 'spirit' is tantamount to calling the earth flat and writing 'Here there be dragons' across it to boot.)

Ancient Man left some tantalizing riddles for us to solve; some of them defy all except the most tortuous of rational explanations but if levitation or, more likely, induced OOBEs were once common to their cultures, the answers are simple. The Glastonbury Zodiac and the Nazcan 'Zoo' are enormous designs ingeniously set out on the land *that can only be seen from the air*. Indeed they were only discovered in modern times by flying over them. Is levitation a lost art? Were the saints and the mediums merely reactivating an ancient practice when they 'flew'? Gravity may not be such a force to be reckoned with, after all.

HOME AND AWAY

Shortly after his experiment with Crookes, Home's tubercular condition became worse. He took his family to the kinder climate of the Mediterranean, where he occasionally gave private seances, but it was evident that his psychical powers were warning, and he retired from the Spiritualist circuit to write his *Lights and Shadows of Spiritualism*, which was published in 1877. In it he was scathing about conjurors masquerading as mediums, or those who eked out a little psychic ability with sleight of hand (or foot). The sceptics reacted with delight: well, he should know if anybody does...

When he lampooned the pathetic and the gullible he was accused of biting the hand that had fed him, and even of taking a sly dig at Mrs Lyons, who so very nearly gave him her fortune:

> I knew once an old lady who, before dining, invariably seated herself at a small table and commenced to tip it. The table was supposed to stand as representative for the spirit of her deceased husband. When the tipping was fairly started, interrogations began. 'Dear Charles, may I eat fish today?' The table would make affirmative motions. 'Thank you, dear Charles, I thought I might, for I felt a strong desire to have fish for dinner.' At times the response was in the negative. Then came something like the following: 'Ah! I thought so, Charles. I felt one of my chills coming on, and fish is bad for me when I have my chills.' I never knew an instance when the answer was not in full unison with her own wishes.

Home died in 1886, already a shadowy figure in the annals of history and, as is the way with those who perform miracles, he was rapidly forgotten except by the hard core of stalwart Spiritualists. (It is significant that the phrase 'nine-days' wonder' describes how short our collective attention span is when faced with the impossible.) Nevertheless, he is still a shining light of integrity compared to the often unscrupulous world of the seance room and the even more sordid magic circle of the sceptics.

In 1871 William Crookes had written this of his researches into psychical phenomena:

Opportunities having since offered for pursuing the investigation, I have gladly availed myself of them for applying to these phenomena careful scientific testing experiments, and I have thus arrived at certain definite results which I think it right should be published. These experiments appear conclusively to establish the existence of a new force, in some unknown manner connected with the human organisation, which for convenience may be called the Psychic Force.

(The 'Psychic Force' was not, of course, 'new' to the human race, but its novelty value was just beginning to appeal to some scientists.)

Three years after this statement, Crookes was given another opportunity to investigate 'the human organization', but this time his reputation was to suffer as a direct result of his involvement with the medium in question. And this time the sceptics were not too hard-pushed to find a word to sum up this downfall. Sex.

2

▫ WHAT KATIE DID ▫

EVEN THE MOST devoted friend of the impossible will find the Crookes-King-Cook collaboration hard to take. Indeed, this case is only for the rarefied appetite of true connoisseurs of bizarre phenomena...

'If facts, their importance cannot be exaggerated – if frauds, their wickedness cannot be exceeded.' E.W. Cox, a contemporary of William Crookes, made these uncompromising comments about the phenomena allegedly induced by the teenage medium Florence Cook who, entranced, produced materializations of a long-dead girl, known as 'Katie King'. These were no vague drifting mists surrounding a floating face, as were many of the so-called materializations of the Victorian seance room, but took the form of a solid young lady in a shroud who walked and talked with the sitters – a spirit made flesh and blood through the mediumship of Florence Cook. Was this, as Spiritualists claimed – and still do – modern proof of the resurrection of the dead? Katie's new body, in which she clothed her spirit, was indeed indistinguishable from that of a living girl – and a very pretty body it was, too, being beautifully set off by her customary white drapings with a fashionably nipped-in waist. Unfortunately, it was also indistinguishable from Florence Cook's.

Katie King has a long history; she first appeared during the initial Spiritualist craze in mid-19th-century America and graced the proceedings of the famous Davenport brothers, William and Ira, whose performances were perhaps no more than stage acts. Reports of Katie's early appearances make her sound like a young Gracie Allen: her voice was shrill 'like that of a person of lower walks of life.' She had an endless supply of chatter, none of which proved the afterlife to have been very educational – but it would be most ungracious to expect the 'living' proof of the resurrection to be loved for her brains as well as her body.

The lovely young ghost had, curiously, adopted 'Katie King' as a *nom d'après vie*, her name when on earth having been Annie Owen Morgan, daughter of the pirate Henry Owen Morgan whose swashbuckling had obviously appealed to Charles II – Morgan had been knighted and became Governor General of Jamaica. He preferred to be known as John King in his new career as a disembodied table-tilter (and notes apparently signed by him have appeared in the SORRAT minilab). Katie, as Annie, had married and borne two children, but she had obviously inherited her father's lax attitude to morality, being a self-confessed liar and a cheat, a thief and murderess all before she died in her early twenties. Her new mission was to prove to the world the truth of Spiritualism in general, and the talents of a few chosen mediums in particular.

COOK AND KING, DYNAMIC DUO

Katie's new lease of life really began when she went into partnership with Eastender Florence Cook in the 1870s, at about the same time that D.D. Home was engaged in experimental work with William Crookes.

Florrie, according to her mother, had always been aware of the presence of spirits. She had heard strange voices and seen shadowy figures since an early age, but her psychic gifts only became spectacular when she was levitated during a table-tilting session with some schoolfriends when she was fifteen. Almost instantly she became the child star of her local Spiritualist circuit, the usual rappings, heavings of furniture, misty lights and so

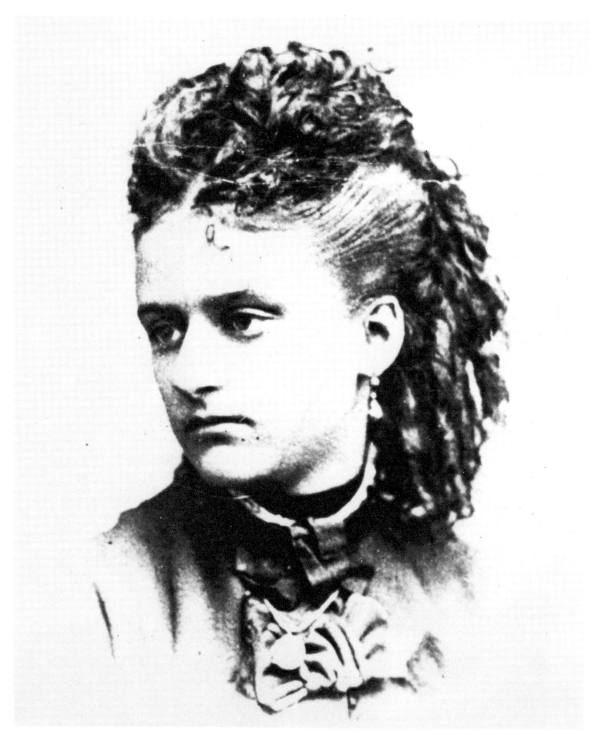

Above Florence Cook, the pert, East-End medium whose greatest claim to fame was the alleged spirit manifestation of a long-dead pirate's daughter, Katie King, while she herself lay entranced in her dimly-lit cabinet. Although Katie and Florrie seemed identical, the spirit said she had been 'much prettier' in life.

Opposite Katie King modestly averts her eye from the camera as she hugs the arm of the distinguished scientist William Crookes. His investigation of Spiritualism began with Home's phenomena, but when Florence Cook offered herself for examination he took to the task with an enthusiasm that laid him open to scandal.

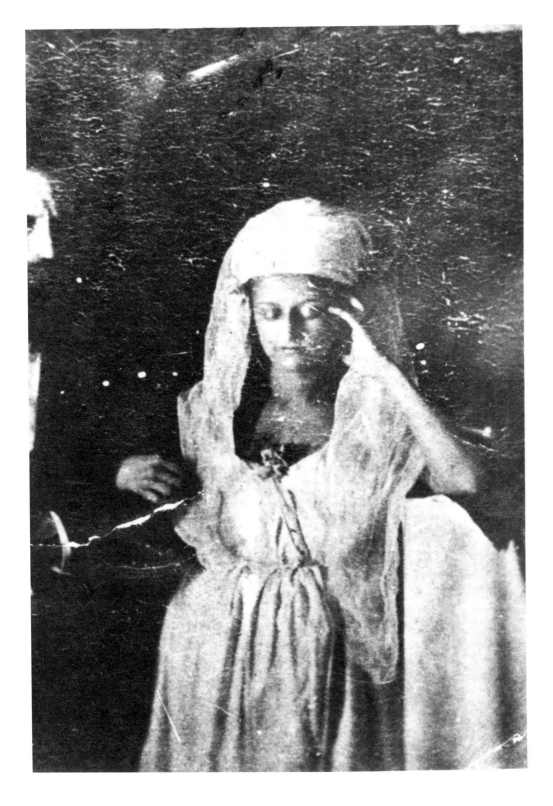

on attending her seances with greater vigour than those that enlivened those of most other mediums. Florrie was particularly adept at 'mirror writing' – scribbles produced when entranced that could only be clearly read reflected in a mirror.

'Automatic' writing is commonly practised by Spiritualists, although with patience anyone can do it to a certain extent. You take a piece of paper and hold a pen in the normal way so that its point rests very gently on the paper. Then you catch your subconscious unawares by distracting it. Think of something else, hold a conversation or watch television. Very probably the pen will begin to twitch and jerk over the paper, scrawling something unintelligible – perhaps just a curly line that could possibly be an attempt at a word. With practice you may well find your pen producing whole sentences, even messages; they are unlikely to be deeply significant ('Take carrots swb phn rasa' is typical – but is it in code? If so, who has the codebook?). Nevertheless, for a few rare people, automatic writing does seem to put them in touch with a profound level of consciousness, but whether of their own mind or someone else's is open to conjecture.

Outside the Spiritualist context there are many recorded instances of the left hand not knowing what the right hand is doing. Emily Brontë's brother Branwell, for example, could write two different letters with both hands simultaneously. (It is tempting to think that had he lived but a few more years his personality and quirky gifts might have made him a passable medium. But he died before the Spiritualist contagion spread to the industrial north, having been claimed by spirits of another sort.)

Florrie's spirit-controlled writing foreswore gibberish and came straight to the point: she was to go to a certain bookseller and there be introduced to the members of the Dalston Association of Spiritualists. Once in their company it was her fate to meet the Editor of *The Spiritualist*, and her future as a famous medium would be assured. All of this came to pass.

Perhaps it is not so amazing that this pretty young girl shot to fame, at least locally, for the spirits had a habit of throwing her up into the air and – on at least one memorable occasion – ripping off her clothes. Florrie is said to have been embarrassed by this incident.

Under the circumstances, Miss Eliza Cliff, in whose Hackney school Florrie worked as assistant teacher, felt she had to dispense with the budding medium's services. The girls were being unsettled by the strange happenings that tended to cluster around Miss Cook, and by the inevitable rumour of even wilder incidents. Their parents were worried that their offspring might become tainted – so Miss Cliff asked Florrie to leave, writing to Mrs Cook: 'I am so grieved at what I am going to write that I can scarcely commence…I am so fond of Florrie and I have such a high opinion of her, that I am sorry to have to say to you that I am compelled to part with her…' Miss Cliff only regretted that Florrie was 'fitted for something far higher and nobler' than Spiritualism. (Almost exactly 100 years later Matthew Manning was asked to leave his boarding school – the other boys were being disturbed by the way the furniture moved around him.)

Then, one night in 1872, a still, white face appeared in the darkness outside the curtains of Florrie's cabinet – the recess that isolates the medium from the sitters and protects her from intrusive rays of light, or prying eyes. This floating mask was announced to be 'Katie King', already a force to be reckoned with across the Atlantic.

By 1873 the Cooks' 'home circle' had achieved fame beyond Hackney, for with the arrival of Katie, nothing less than a miracle was being regularly enacted; the resurrection of the body, the corruptible having put on incorruptible, faith made flesh.

Florrie, like many another medium before and since, preferred to go into her trances behind a cabinet in which her psychic energies could build up. After a while – thirty minutes seemed to be the longest the sitters had to wait – the curtain would be drawn back and a figure, all in white, would emerge, while Florrie continued to lie slumped in the cabinet. Katie then walked among the guests, exchanging small talk (her voice was no longer shrill as it was in her American manifestations, but her conversation still left a lot to be desired). She was fond of touching them and encouraging them to feel for themselves that she was truly flesh and blood. When her allotted time was up, Katie would prettily make her excuses and return behind the curtain. In a few minutes Florrie would reappear, having surfaced from her trance – and Katie presumably, had returned to the nebulous world from whence she came.

ECTOPLASM IN UNDERCLOTHES

The theory was that the medium's trance enabled her to exude a misty white substance that the spirit moulded into a temporary body. This 'ectoplasm' was rarely actually seen building up by sitters at Florrie's seances, as the transformation happened discreetly behind the curtain, but its existence was attested at other gatherings for many years. It is still said to appear today, but only at very private meetings, well away from sceptical eyes.

There are two types of recorded mediumship: 'mental', where the medium produces information, often purporting to come from deceased relatives of the sitters, that she (most mediums are women) could not have discovered by normal means; and 'physical', where the medium's powers directly affect inanimate objects or produce them from thin air (where they are called 'apports'), or in extreme cases produce manifestations of the dead. Home, although mainly a physical medium, had often had flashes of genuine clairvoyance; Florrie was exclusively physical.

Ectoplasm is an odd, elusive substance – indeed, some sceptics refute its very existence, and even among those who claim to have seen it, it can appear totally repulsive. Florrie's delicate white clouds that gradually took human form were disconcerting, but not sickening, as are the reports of thick, clotted, mucus-like

substances that have been observed to flow from every bodily orifice of other mediums. (The sheer nastiness of ectoplasm is graphically lampooned in *Ghostbusters*. Two of our intrepid trio of parapsychologists are enthusiastic about the mess of 'ectoplasmic residue' left oozing and dripping in the wake of a phantom. But Dr Yateman is not impressed. 'Someone blows their nose and you want to keep it?' he asks in disgust.)

Brian Inglis, staunch champion of the paranormal, says in *The Hidden Power* (1986):

> Ectoplasm, after all, has sometimes been reported as visible and tangible...Geley [a foremost psychical researcher in the 1920s] made the daring suggestion that ectoplasm may turn out to be the basic stuff from which animal matter is constructed. If so, the evolutionary programme may have endowed humanity with the potential ability to create entities and give them a semblance of life.

Sometimes the ectoplasmic filaments do not give substance to a spirit, like Katie King, but content themselves with becoming 'pseudopods' or telescopic antennae, that are extruded from the medium's body and can move furniture, or even levitate the sitters. Perhaps when invisible it is they that tilt tables, or aim the crockery during poltergeist attacks? Was it a tightrope of ectoplasmic twine that got D.D. Home from window to window at Ashley House, Westminster on that memorable night?

The trouble with ectoplasm is that it has so few friends. In theory, its existence makes perfect sense even if, or perhaps especially when, that theory is carried to extremes, as with Geley's idea given above. In practice even would-be believers find themselves echoing Harry Houdini's contemptuous statement: 'Nothing has crossed my path to make me think that the Great Almighty will allow emanations from the human body of such horrible, revolting, vicious shapes, which like "genii from the bronze bottle" ring bells, move handkerchiefs, wobble tables and do other "flap-

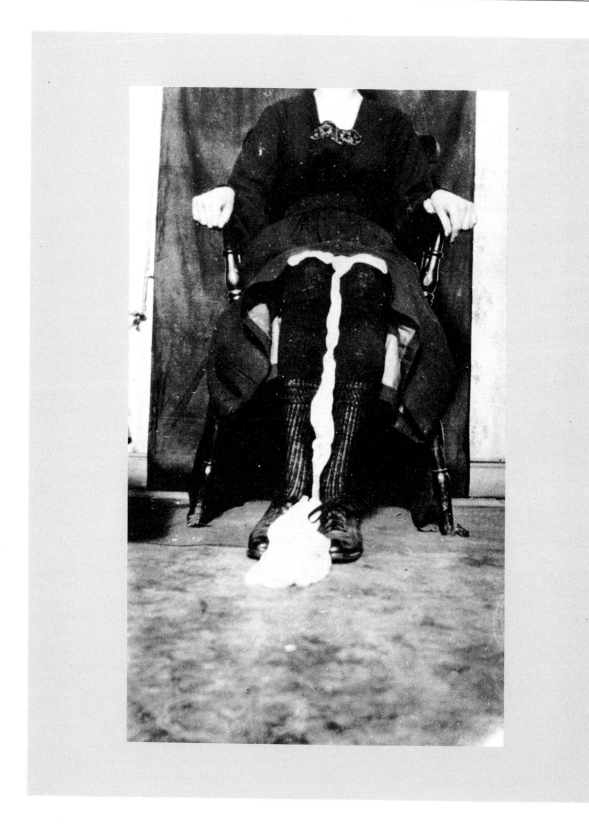

doodle" stunts.' Houdini was, of course, an infamous sceptic towards the end of his life.

In answer to my own questions about personal views of ectoplasm, one senior member of the Society for Psychical Research (who is not known to be particularly tainted with the creeping horror of the paranormal that affects so much of its membership) said 'it's butter muslin. It always has been and always will be...I did see some produced in a seance once. It smelt appallingly of B.O. which wasn't surprising, considering where it was kept'.

So on the one hand ectoplasm is God's clay from which all living things are, and can be fashioned, or a disgusting secretion (usually fraudulent at that) with which to con gullible members of the public. It is hard to imagine two opposing beliefs that encompass the noble and the obscene so totally. But from believers and sceptics alike at least there are no reports that Katie King was in any way repulsive – if anything, quite the reverse.

If the theory is true that making sudden grabs for entranced mediums is dangerous for their health, then on at least one occasion Florence Cook had a lucky escape.

On the evening of 9 December 1873, one of the sitters at the Cook home circle was a Mr William Volckman. As casual callers were not encouraged he must have been a welcome guest, having received one of the Cooks' handwritten invitations that bore the warning 'make no enquiries'. But as the seance got underway and Katie duly appeared in their midst he grew increasingly irritated by the 'obvious' similarities between medium and materialization. They were, he concluded, the same girl, and an outrageous trick was being played on them all. In a fit of fury he leapt up and grabbed Katie, trying to hold on to the wriggling phantom by her very solid waist.

Among the other sitters there was horror and consternation. The Earl and Countess of Caithness and the barrister Henry Dumphy were present; all were friends of the Cooks and aware of the dangers allegedly inherent in such rash action. They seized the heretic Volckman and a scuffle ensued that ended with part of his beard being pulled out by the roots. During the fracas, Katie had disappeared; Dumphy stated later that she had dissolved from the feet upwards, making a movement 'similar to that of a seal in water'. (During Home's seances solid-feeling hands and arms had also dissolved at the touch of the sitters.)

Determined to follow up his assault, Volckman rushed to the cabinet, where he found no trace of Katie, but only Florrie, lying in her customary entranced state – but a little dishevelled. The struggle with the other guests had lost him about five minutes of valuable time, in which, he was convinced, he could have discovered Katie shedding her white frock to become Florrie. Yet Florrie was still bound with sealed tape, (this voluntary bondage of mediums before seances was taken to be a sign of their good faith).

Significantly, however, shortly after this incident Mr Volckman became the husband of another famous London medium, Mrs Samuel Guppy, who was known to be wildly jealous of Florrie/Katie. Florrie, meanwhile, suffered a slight reversal of fortune in the following months. She and her sisters (who also professed to have mediumistic gifts) had been paid a retainer by a rich old man, Charles Blackburn, to give him private sittings – presumably in the hope that he and his mentally sick daughter Eliza would glean a little spiritual comfort from them. But the Volckman incident had gained the Cooks some unwelcome notoriety, about which Mr Blackburn had grave doubts,

The Belfast medium, Kathleen Golligher, produces a stream of ectoplasm under experimental conditions. This strange, and some would say disgusting, substance once enjoyed a vogue at the seances of 'physical' mediums, where the spirits allegedly used it to shape materializations of the dead, or as rods or levers with which to tilt or levitate furniture. Even if genuine, does ectoplasm provide proof of an afterlife, or is it yet one more example of the unacceptable face of Spiritualism?

and he even threatened to stop paying their retainer.

Hearing that William Crookes was currently investigating Home, Florrie hastened to add her contribution to psychical research. Crookes was ingenuously delighted to investigate the now famous Cook-King partnership first hand. It was from that moment that his problems really began.

Crookes announced his programme of psychical investigation with Florence Cook, not in any scientific journal, nor even in a quality newspaper, but in *The Spiritualist*. If, as some commentators have suggested, this was designed to restore the public's faith in Florrie after Katie had been almost literally floored by Mrs Guppy's fiancé, then it was ridiculously ill-placed. Spiritualists still believed in her anyway – why preach to the converted?

And so his work with Florrie began. It seemed more convenient for her, and occasionally her mother and sisters, to move in with the Crookes at Mornington Road in north-west London. Mrs Crookes was in the house but not often much in evidence, for she was expecting their tenth child at the time and was often confined to her room.

The first time Crookes had seen Florrie and Katie together was when Florrie approached him about the possibility of their collaboration, and he visited the Cook family home at Hackney. Katie had appeared from behind the curtain and asked him to accompany her into the curtained-off recess, using only a phosphorus lamp to light the way. Once inside the cabinet, he relates:

> Kneeling down, I let air into the lamp, and by its light I saw the young lady dressed in black velvet, as she had been in the early part of the evening, and to all appearance perfectly senseless; she did not move when I took her hand and held the light quite close to her face, but continued quietly breathing. Raising the lamp, I looked around and saw Katie standing close behind Miss Cook. She was robed in flowing white drapery as we had seen her previously during the seance.

> Holding one of Miss Cook's hands in mine and still kneeling, I passed the lamp up and down so as to illuminate Katie's whole figure, and satisfy myself thoroughly that I was really looking at the veritable Katie whom I had clasped in my arms a few minutes before, and not at the phantasm of a disordered brain. She did not speak, but moved her head in recognition. Three separate times did I carefully examine Miss Cook crouching before me, to be sure that the hand I held was that of a living woman, and three separate times did I turn the lamp to Katie and examine her with steadfast scrutiny until I had no doubt whatever of her objective reality.

The Reverend Charles Davies, a shrewd psychical researcher with time on his hands, spent a full three hours with Katie, whom he witnessed materializing in good light. The spirit girl had:

> ...allowed me to go up to the cupboard and touch her face and hand, after first putting to me the pertinent question, 'do you squeeze?' On assuring her I did not do anything so improper, the manipulations were permitted...I should like to submit these particulars to a dispassionate jury for them to decide whether I was really for those three hours in direct contact with supernatural beings or simply taken in by one of the most satisfactory 'physical' mediums it was ever my good fortune to meet.

Of course not all sitters were ready to believe the two women were separate beings, and had insisted that extreme measures be taken to prevent Florrie playing tricks.

Customarily, before the seance began, Florrie was bound with a cord which was then sealed by one of the sitters – both cord and seal were always found intact at the end of the materialization. And although the indignities commonly inflicted on mediums of a later date, such as filling their mouths with fruit juice to prevent ventriloquism and examining *all* their orifices for hidden 'ectoplasm', were not practised on Florrie, on at least one occa-

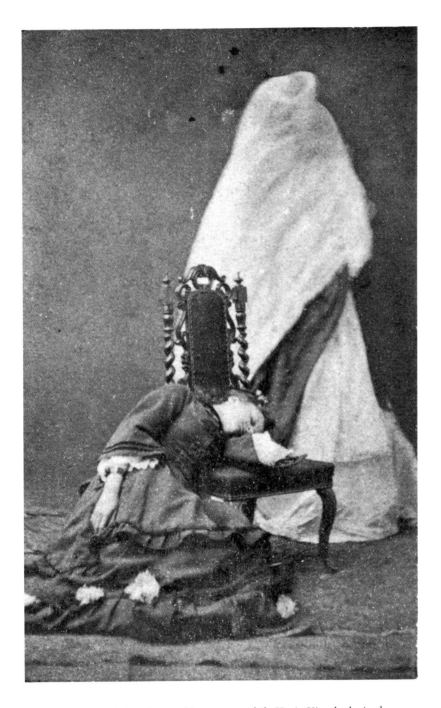

Florrie Cook lies slumped in trance, while Katie King lurks in the
background. One of over forty photographs taken of the Cook-King
partnership by William Crookes while the medium lived in his house,
this was intended to prove that girl and ghost were separate entities.
Unfortunately Katie's features are obscured by ectoplasmic mists.

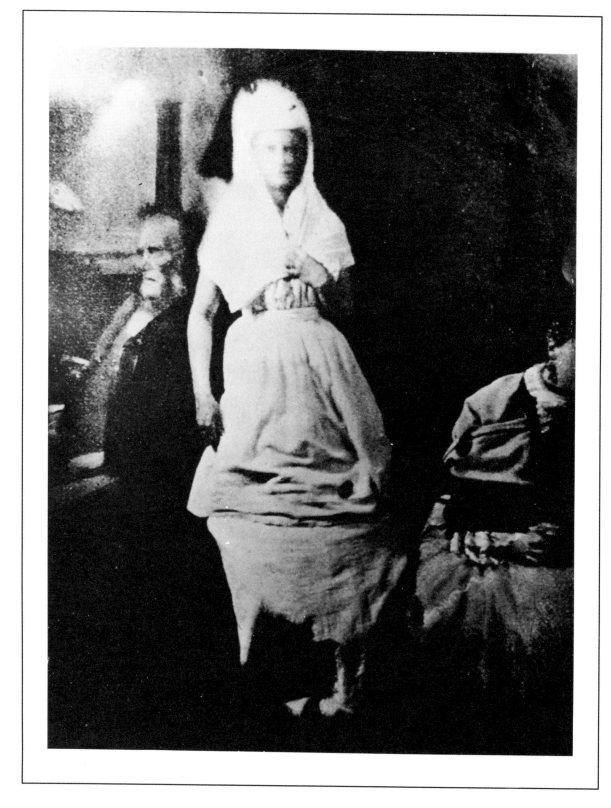

sion her hair was actually nailed to the floor where she lay. Katie still appeared.

KATIE: THE LIVING IMAGE?

But the physical similarities between the two young women, one alive and one dead, continued to cause comment and still does. Certainly the photographs taken by Crookes show Katie and Florrie to be identical, except for their clothes, and those that purported to prove their separate existence show only Katie in her flowing robes and someone (in one case, half a someone) in a black dress sitting next to her, or Florrie slumped in front of a tall white figure with some veil-like material blowing across its face. As 'proof' it seems sad to the point of being risible.

Of the individual photographs, one shows Crookes arm-in-arm with Katie, looking tenderly at her – or perhaps his concern is for the emergence of some dark material at her bosom and upper arm...was Katie wearing Florrie's black dress under her shroud? Another, very strange, photograph shows a blurred Katie staring straight into the lens immediately in front of a sitter, who stares resolutely to his right, almost as if she isn't there, or he isn't. (The problem is resolved when one realizes that we are seeing his reflection. Is this truly Looking Glass land?) The most peculiar thing about this picture is that Katie is kneeling, or so it seems, on some article of furniture covered over to look like an extension of her dress; after all Katie *was* said to be 10 cm (4 in) taller than her medium. The illusion of the extra

One of the more bizarre photographs of the Katie King seances. The gentleman on the left, who seems to be in the grip of a catatonic trance, is in fact a reflection in a mirror. The medium, cut in half by Crookes' oddly inept photography, must be assumed to be Florrie Cook (although sceptics suggest that her sister or other accomplice took on the role from time to time). Katie herself appears to be uncomfortably balanced on a stool or small table, with her elegant shroud draped over it. The spirit was said, after all, to be taller than her medium.

height was badly stage-managed, her dress is obviously bunched up at her knees and her legs appear ridiculously long.

But who was this incompetent stage manager?

Doubts about the Crookes-Cook alliance grow when one realizes that even these ludicrous photographs were obviously the best of a peculiar bunch; of the fifty-five photographs taken of Katie and Florrie by Crookes only a few survive; he destroyed the rest, together with their negatives, shortly before his death in 1919.

Crookes used five cameras, two of them stereoscopic, operating simultaneously during these bizarre photographic sessions. Because of the injurious effect of the flashlight on entranced mediums, Florrie's head was swathed in a shawl, thus playing yet again right into the hands of the sceptics. Crookes recorded that:

> It was a common thing for the seven or eight of us in the laboratory to see Miss Cook and Katie at the same time, under the blaze of electric light...we did not on these occasions see the face of the medium because of the shawl but we saw her hands and feet: we saw her move uneasily under the influence of the intense light, and we heard her moan occasionally. I have one photograph of the two together, but Katie is seated in front of Miss Cook's head.

Protruding hands and feet, uneasy tossings and turnings and the odd moan do not add up to the proverbial can of beans as evidence. From a layman this statement would be taken with a pinch of salt, from a scientist of Crookes' training and standing not all the salt in Siberia could sway the critics. Arrogant though he may have been in his assumption that he, of all people, would be believed, Crookes deserves more than our pity, or even a knowing nudge and wink.

Friends of the impossible should know

better than to dismiss out of hand what seems to be a blatant fraud. And perhaps the most relevant question *we* should be asking is: did Crookes himself really believe in Katie? It is worth quoting his defence in full:

> Every test I have proposed she had at once agreed to submit to with the utmost willingness; she is open and straightforward in speech, and I have never seen anything approaching the slightest symptom of a wish to deceive. Indeed, I do not believe she could carry on a deception if she were to try, and if she did she would certainly be found out very quickly, for such a line of action is altogether foreign to her nature. And to imagine that an innocent schoolgirl of 15 should be able to conceive and then successfully carry out for three years so gigantic an imposture as this, and in that time submit to any test which might be imposed on her, should bear the strictest scrutiny, should be willing to be searched at any time, either before or after a seance, and should meet with even better success in my own house than that of her parents, knowing that she visited me with the express object of submitting to strict scientific tests – to imagine, I say, the Katie King of the last three years to be the result of imposture does more violence to one's reason and common sense than to believe her to be what she herself affirms.

Does the gentleman protest too much?

But Katie was flighty, like all the Cosmic Joker's creatures. At precisely the same time as she was materializing through Florrie in Mornington Road, she was also appearing at seances in Philadelphia. We know so little about the spirit world that this Spiritualist schizophrenia may come easily to the likes of Katie. But Crookes was furious, to him there was only *Florrie's* Katie. When shown a photograph alleging to be her American twin he had no hesitation in denouncing it as a fraud.

Katie looked like Florrie simply because

that's who she was, claim the sceptics, and on the surface the case looks black against Crookes. It is simply not good enough to cite his stature as a scientist and his integrity in previous, and later, years, as his champions still do. They even assert that it is impossible to believe that his infatuation with Katie was sexual, and that he could never have considered conducting a liaison with Florrie/Katie because his wife was in the house at the time. This is extraordinarily naive; this might even have added spice to the situation. Men of repute and integrity have fallen in love and made fools of themselves before and since and many have been duped by the simplest, and most brazen frauds – such as Sir Arthur Conan Doyle in the case of the Cottingley Fairies (page 90).

There are three possible explanations for the Crookes-Cook-King collaboration: one, that the scientist had behaved scandalously in his private and professional life by having an affair with Florrie under his wife's nose, and at the same time colluding with the medium to manufacture fraudulent results of his investigation into 'Katie King'. An alternative is that he was, indeed, besotted with Florrie – and therefore her lookalike Katie – but kept up the pretence, even to her, that he believed her outrageous 'act' to save his face and keep her close to him. The third option is that, against all odds, she was genuine, he was genuine, all of it was genuine.

Although Crookes had behaved strangely for a man with a scientist's high regard for detail – omitting names and addresses of other witnesses of the Katie King phenomenon from his records, for example – this may have been due to excessive regard for Florrie's own quaint rules ('make no enquiries'). Unfortunately this paucity of information about the sitters has meant that few other eye-witness accounts have come down to us.

However, one prime witness was Mrs Ross-Church, better known as the novelist Florence Marryat, who gives a vivid account of seeing the girl and ghost separately in *There is no death*:

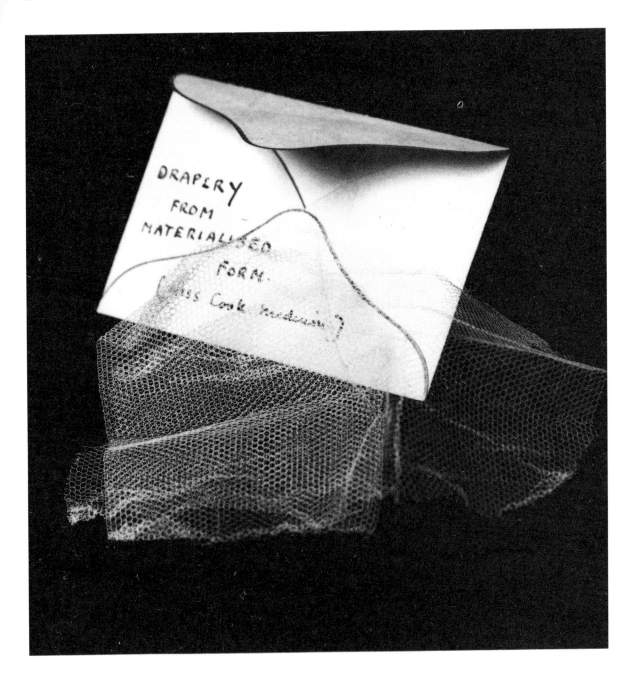

A piece of stiff gauze, said to have been materialized by Florence Cook,
carefully preserved by rival medium Mrs Guppy. Fake ectoplasm was
often discovered to be regurgitated butter muslin, which proved more
about the mediums' muscle control than about the hereafter.
If the dead can be created and clothed in ectoplasm in the seance room
then surely more mundane manifestations – such as pieces of gauze – can
also be summoned up. Unfortunately, such museum pieces do not in
themselves constitute proof of genuine phenomena.

Sometimes Katie resembled Florence Cook in features; at others she was totally different. One evening Katie walked out and perched herself on my knee. I could feel that she was much plumper and heavier than Miss Cook, but on this occasion she resembled her in features, and I told her so.

Katie did not seem to consider this a compliment, and said: 'I know I am, I can't help it, but I was much prettier than that in earth life. You shall see, some day. You shall see.' After she had retired that evening she put her head out of the curtain and said: 'I want to see Mrs Ross-Church.' I rose and went to her, and she pulled me inside the curtain, which I found was so thin that the gas from the other room made everything quite visible. Katie pulled my dress impatiently and said: 'Sit down on the ground', which I did. She then sat on my lap. Florence Cook meanwhile was lying on the floor in a deep trance. Katie seemed very anxious that I should ascertain that it was Florrie. 'Touch her,' she said: 'take her hand, pull her curls. Do you see that it is Florrie lying there?' When I assured her that I was quite satisfied there was no doubt of it, the spirit said: 'Then look round this way and see what I looked like in earth life.'

I turned to the form in my arms, and it was my amazement to see a woman, fair as the day, with large grey or blue eyes, a white skin and a profusion of golden red hair. Katie enjoyed my surprise, and then asked: 'Am I not prettier than Florrie now?' She then gave me a lock of her own hair and a lock of Florence Cook's. Florrie's is almost black, soft and silky; Katie's a coarse golden red.

Crookes had noted some precise differences between the two girls; Katie was taller, heavier and broader in the face, with a much fairer complexion, and longer fingers. Florrie had pierced ears, Katie had not. On one occasion the medium had a large blister on her neck but when Katie materialized, her neck was fair and smooth as usual. Astonishingly, he took no comparative photographs of the girls' pierced and unpierced ears or the respective length of

their fingers, or if he did there is no known record of them. Even with fairly primitive photography it was possible to give some indication of the size of hands and fingers, for example. We do not even know by how much of a sliver of an inch Katie's fingers exceeded Florrie's, and possibly most people couldn't care less, but the fact remains that the man was a scientist allegedly investigating the most epoch-making phenomenon since Christ's resurrection. What was he thinking of?

PLAYING A GAME OF LADIES' DOUBLES

An even more damning aspect of this case is the part played by another young medium, Mary Showers, who stayed with the Crookes briefly during the Cooks' residence. She performed a double act with Florrie, both girls sinking simultaneously into trances behind the curtain and, after a short while, two materializations appeared arm-in-arm: Katie and 'Florence Maple', who bore a more than passing resemblance to Mary. Crookes later acknowledged that Mary had confessed herself a fraud, so why did Katie align herself with a blatant fake if she, too, were not guilty? Already unsavoury, the story becomes grotesque.

To the worldly-wise eyes of the late-twentieth century, most of the witnesses' accounts of Katie's manifestations contain some clues about her nature, and they do not point to much that is notably spiritual. Katie was a flirt, a tease and an exhibitionist to both sexes, flouncing around Crookes' semi-darkened laboratory, sitting on laps, touching and being

Katie King having her pulse taken by one Dr Gully of Malvern at a seance in William Crookes' north London home. It was found to be faster than her medium's, but sceptics point out that the effect might be achieved simply by Florrie's rushing to don Katie's robes. The shroud is curiously bunched at the knee, as if forced over the widest point of a crinoline, but Katie, throughout her liason with Florrie, showed a particularly keen dress sense.

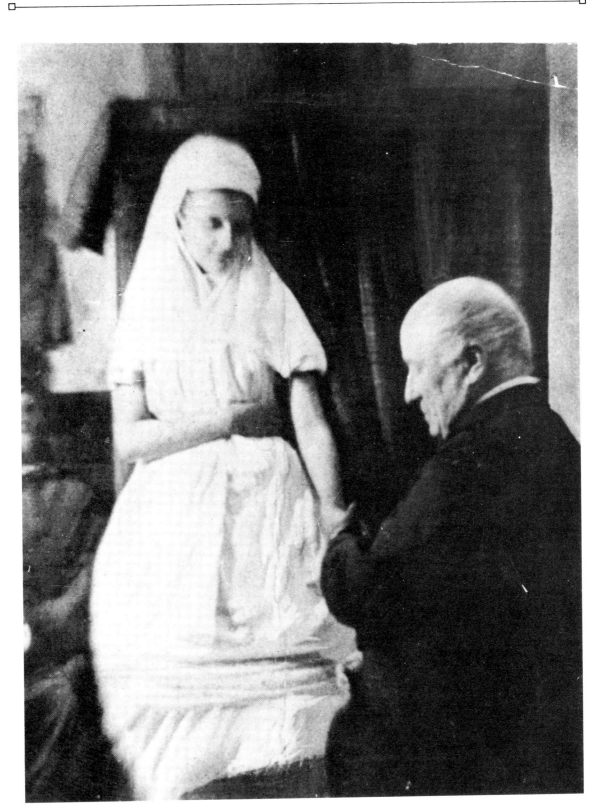

touched and on one occasion, even stepping naked out of her designer shroud. 'Now,' she said, 'you can see that I am a woman.' And, as Mrs Ross-Church admitted, she was 'a most beautifully made woman too.'

Even being photographed arm-in-arm with Crookes seems today a curious procedure. Could he not have demonstrated her tangibility in some less questionable fashion, by standing her on the scales perhaps? In the 1870s even a kiss was deemed a profoundly intimate act, and to stand arm-in-arm with a pert young lady implies somewhat more than a scientist-subject relationship. Perhaps Crookes believed it to look protective and avuncular; poor Crookes. (Nevertheless he had the common sense to withhold this photograph from public circulation during his lifetime, believing it would have been misunderstood. He was right.)

Even to have proved beyond question that Florrie and Katie were distinctly different girls meant little, for Florrie's sister Kate also took up residence in Mornington Road, and if Mary Showers knew the house well enough to produce her 'materialization act', perhaps she too had been there before. Either girl could have acted as a stand-in for Florrie, dressed in black, while she donned a white robe and flitted around in the gloaming. Katie's shroud was on occasion extraordinarily voluminous as if it covered another dress and many petticoats, which would partly explain why Katie was said to be a heavier girl than Florrie; it is easier to become heavier than lighter, after all.

Those few surviving photographs of Katie show her to be fickle in her choice of body; when arm-in-arm with Crookes and modestly averting her gaze from the camera she seems short-waisted with a thick torso and wide face, when apparently kneeling precariously on the small table she is slim, with a fashionably tiny waist. When having her pulse taken by one Dr Gully of Malvern (it was faster than Florrie's, and rushing to don white raiment would have had such an effect) she looks plump, and again her skirt is peculiarly bloated as if hiding a multitude of sins.

Katie had announced that she was available on earth for a limited period only; in 1875 that time was rapidly running out. Crookes tells of the affecting scene he witnessed as she said an emotional farewell to her friend, medium and double, Florrie:

> After closing the curtain she conversed with me for some time, and then walked across the room where Miss Cook was lying senseless on the floor. Stooping over her, Katie touched her, and said, 'Wake up Florrie, wake up! I must leave you now.' Miss Cook then woke and tearfully entreated Katie to stay a little time longer. 'My dear, I can't; my work is done. God bless you,' Katie replied, and then continued speaking to Miss Cook.
>
> For several minutes the two were conversing with each other, till at last Miss Cook's tears prevented her speaking. Following Katie's instructions I then came forward to support Miss Cook, who was falling on to the floor, sobbing hysterically. I looked round, but the white-robed Katie had gone.

There is a theatrical saying: 'a conjuror's best assistant is Miss Direction'. Could Miss Cook's pretty hysterics have covered for the final exit of the woman in white?

With Katie recalled to the unknown, there was no point in Florrie staying on for further investigation, especially as she then told Crookes that she had, unbeknown to him, been married for a couple of months. The lucky man was a sailor, Edward Corner, with whom she was spliced at the end of April, 1874, but she had thought it best not to mention this to Crookes while living in his house. Meanwhile her sister Kate had become medium-in-residence at old Mr Blackburn's, materializing as 'Lillie Gordon', who wrote him affectionate pencilled notes – to which he replied with 'love and kisses' – when he became bed-ridden. After his death all the Cooks (except for Florrie), and

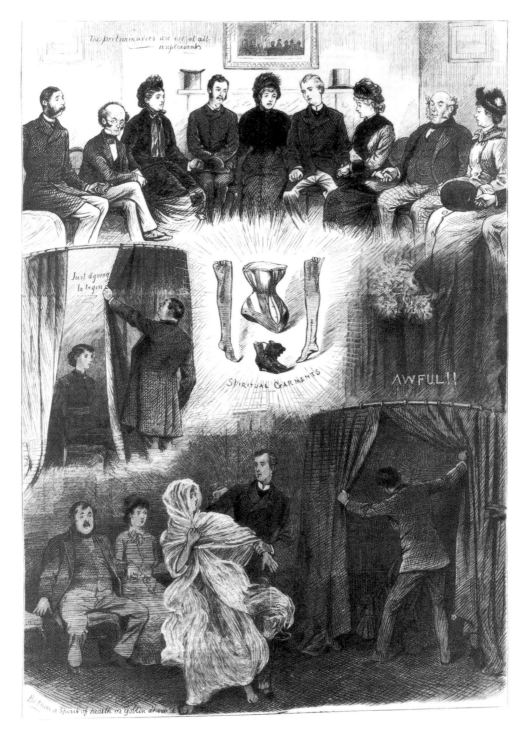

Six years after Katie King returned to the spirit world, her medium,
Florence Cook, materialized a young girl known as 'Marie', who
entertained the sitters by singing and dancing. On one occasion, however,
Sir George Sitwell grabbed the spirit – and found he held Florence Cook
in his arms, attired only in her underwear. This incident marked the end of
her career as a medium.

Captain Corner, benefited by his will. They had all given him much comfort.

Six years after Katie's departure Florrie was giving another seance to a distinguished audience. These days her spirit partner was a young manifestation called Marie, who provided more in the way of entertainment than Katie (who admittedly occasionally stripped naked), in that she sang and did a few pretty dance steps. There was something about this Marie, however...One of the sitters, Sir George Sitwell, could stand this travesty no longer; he seized Marie while others flooded the seance room with light. This was to be no Volckman debacle. He held on tight and was not surprised to discover he held Florrie, attired only in her underwear.

Florrie sank into relative obscurity as a middle-class housewife in Usk Vale, Monmouthshire. It was there that she was called upon in 1893 by one Francis Anderson, whom she promptly seduced, gaily telling tales of the good old days when she performed her 'materialization trick' for William Crookes, with whom she had also had an affair. The whole 'investigation' was a cover for their passion, and her silence about her marriage a shrewd expedient – for Mr Blackburn was threatening to cut off her retainer after the Volckman incident. Anderson, confessing all to the Society for Psychical Research in 1922, described the Corners' house minutely, and with relish: 'I can remember the scene of how it all started as if I saw it now.' But when his memory was put to the test it seemed as if he had been describing a completely different house. So how could any of his testimony be trusted, so long after the event? But surely it's easy to muddle bricks and mortar, while the memory of having an affair with the infamous Florrie Corner (née Cook) is less likely to become confused...

William Crookes had been hurt by the overwhelming scepticism with which his fellow scientists had received the results of his investigations, and gave up active psychical research, although he was to remain its staunch champion to the end of his life. He was

knighted twenty years after his work with Florrie. During his long and distinguished career he discovered the element thallium, and his experiments with vacuums were to lead to the invention of the cathode ray tube and X-rays.

In his presidential address to the British Association in 1898 he told his fellow scientists: 'Thirty years have passed since I published an account of experiments tending to show that outside our scientific knowledge there exists a Force exercised by intelligence differing from the ordinary intelligence common to mortals. I have nothing to retract. I adhere to my already published statements. Indeed, I might add much thereto.'

If we are to take his 'thirty years ago' literally then he cannot be referring to Florrie, whose talents he investigated only twenty-four years before. Even if taken as poetic licence, the statement could just as well be referring to his work with D.D. Home – perhaps far better if it were.

Florrie's flouncings were destined to make uneasy history; like Katie, although dead they won't lie down. Devoted and unquestioning Spiritualists naturally believe that Florrie is little short of a martyr to the cause and Crookes much maligned. Sceptics (of whom there are a great many) find everything about the whole story phoney. It is an insult to our intelligence.

But students of the impossible know a double bluff when they see one.

The plaster and lath cosmic fakery, the vulgar buffoonery, the red nose and baggy trousers in the endless tragi-comedy of Spiritualism hides an act that is hard to follow. The central part may have overwhelmed the little girl from Hackney – the Joker wrote her out but she carried on stumbling through the part that made her famous – but then it wasn't created exclusively for her. Whether or not Katie King really lived and died on earth, she won't go away; in 1930 she appeared at Dr Glen Hamilton's seance in Winnipeg, and –

perhaps to celebrate the centenary of her controversial relationship with William Crookes – she appeared in Rome, (looking Italian) in 1974, through the mediumship of Fulvio Rendhell. She will be back, true to form, bearing a striking resemblance to her medium, or a pop star or princess or a face on a cornflake packet. She will elude your grasp and photographs of her will look like cardboard cut-outs or her medium or ... Make no mistake, What Katie Did Next is a chapter not yet finished.

A RAG, A BONE, A HANK OF HAIR

Even among Christians, whose creed alleges their belief in the resurrection of the body, full form materializations of the dead are treated with disbelief or horror. Spiritualism in general has found no favour with orthodox Christianity; where if it is not fake it is blasphemy, and usually both. Katie certainly is past praying for in their eyes (and, of course, a good many others'). Even if she were not Florrie draped in a sheet, if she were really from beyond the grave, surely she must be conjured up through some dark practices, some devilish sorcery?

The occult, the black arts, traditionally include the practice of necromancy – the raising of the dead in order to prophesy the future, like some hideous speaking-doll wound up by the magician. At least Katie carried with her no taint of physical corruption – her shroud was clean, and although it was only right to treat her with caution, rubber gloves and disinfectant were not required. The dead produced by the great Brazilian medium, Mirabelli, were often much more disturbing.

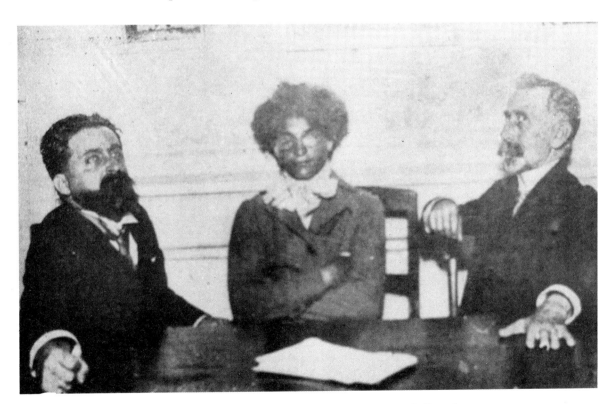

A dead poet materializes between the medium Mirabelli and an understandably perturbed sitter. Mirabelli's materializations sometimes stank of putrefaction, thus raising questions about the nature of his powers and their similarities with necromancy.

At his seances, which were held in all degrees of light, skeletons would build up in the air, clothed with ragged flesh and stinking of decay. At his most successful, he produced solid human beings, which (unlike Katie) bore absolutely no resemblance to their medium – in one case the man he conjured out of nothing was clearly of African origin, as the photographs taken at the time show. (His remarkable appearance would certainly have caused comment if he had been seen around São Paulo, whiling away the time between fake seances.) On another occasion, which was also caught on camera, a dead poet materialized between Mirabelli and a sitter – who not unnaturally is rigid with fear, showing the whites of his eyes like a terrified horse. The phenomenon may be genuine, but is it nice?

Undoubtedly Carmine Mirabelli was possessed of extraordinary powers. A leading light in the Brazilian Spiritist movement (which followed the French medium Alan Kardec) Mirabelli exhibited paranormal gifts that put him at least on a par with Home. He levitated, and on one occasion he began the seance handcuffed; as he rose into the air he dematerialized, leaving the handcuffs to clatter on the floor. He was discovered elsewhere in the house behind a locked door.

Mirabelli produced an astonishing range of phenomena: automatic writing and speaking in tongues (up to thirty known languages were reported); clear demonstrations of prophecy, telepathy and phenomena usually associated with poltergeists; the teleportation of objects and even of people; mysterious fires that suddenly started up and quenched themselves; smashing crockery and the apparent molecular changes of solid objects. A fan began wriggling, and when a skull that Mirabelli merely looked at began to move, the psychiatrist Dr Franco da Rocha noted: 'When I picked up the skull, I felt something strange in my hands, something fluid, as if a globular liquid were touching my palm. When I concentrated my attention further, I saw something similar to an irradiation pass over the skull as when you rapidly expose a mirror to luminous

rays.' His colleague, Dr Felipe Ache, hazarded that Mirabelli's strange gifts were 'the result of the radiation of nervous forces that we all have but that Mirabelli has in extraordinary excess.'

But have we all the ability, to a greater or lesser extent, to produce the spectacular physical manifestations that brought with them such pungent reminders of the grave? And if we have it, do we want it? (Like the question: 'Do you sincerely want to be rich?', with its implication that if you sincerely did then you would be, the question: 'Do you sincerely want to be psychic?' is similarly loaded. There are relatively few rich people in the world and even fewer great psychics. Like the self-made millionaire, the Homes and the Gellers are there to show us it can be done but perhaps not by us. Not today, thank you.)

Raising the dead in a physical form is inevitably a queasy business; few phenomena offend the Great Conspirators more than the apparent control of the dead by the living. And, although millions subscribe to a belief in some sort of afterlife it is usually envisaged as a *spiritual* existence, a pristine progress of the soul.

We make sure our dead decompose in the decent privacy of the grave, or are consumed by fire as soon as possible. Hygiene is not the real reason for the precautions: there are few terrors more basic than being stalked by a mass of corruption. All children's nightmares are B movies by Hammer Films; even before they are sure what they are, children are frightened of skeletons.

Scourge of the seance room, William Marriott, with some of the tricks of the trade, pathetically obvious in daylight, but cleverly lit in the gloaming of a believer's parlour they could take on the identity of the departed. Such flim-flammery has given mediumship a bad reputation and while often deserved, some rare exponents produce spectacular phenomena for which there is no everyday explanation. Paranormal phenomena tend to tease; the more they are sought, expecially by sceptics, the more elusive they become. Yet they flourish in an atmosphere of belief and encouragement, to the delight of sceptics.

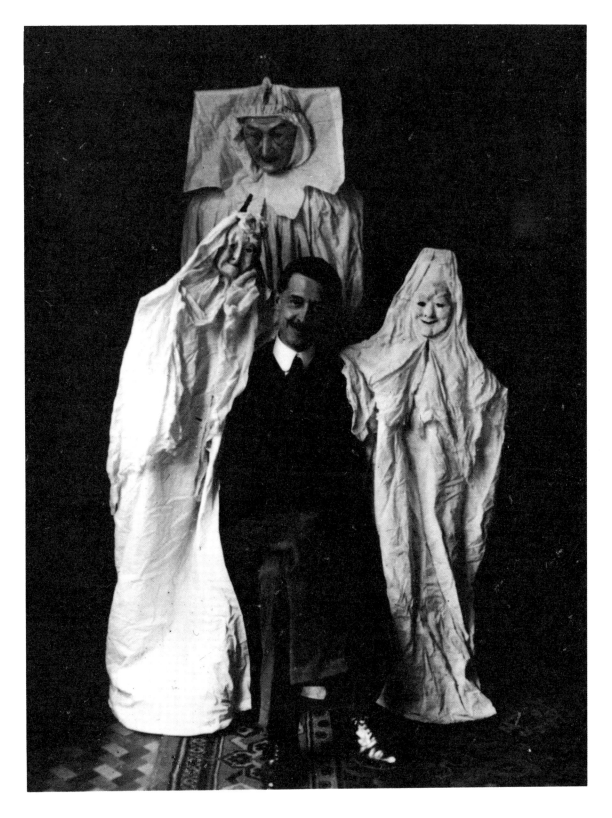

On that sinister island, Haiti, the dead have to be held down under elaborate, and very heavy, stone slabs or walled up in solid mausoleums, for otherwise they would fall prey to sorcerers (who proliferate in the voodoo-ridden culture) and be turned into the living dead – zombies.

The sorcerer's aim is to make cheap labour out of the re-animated corpses over which he casts a spell. They inhabit a twilight world with no memory of their immediate past and no knowledge of their death. They see with the unfocused eyes of the dead; their faces are blank; they speak rarely, and then only with the nasal twang associated in Haiti with death cults. Zombies can eat but cannot touch meat or salt; if they put either in their mouths they will wake up to their nightmare situation and seek out their graves, falling upon them in despair and horror, only to turn into a mass of putrefaction.

In the 1930s an American journalist, Zora Hurston, visited Haiti and was, not unnaturally, incredulous at the zombie stories that abounded. When the opportunity came her way to see an alleged zombie in the flesh she lost no time in seeing the phenomenon for herself. The story was a poignant one: in 1907 a local woman, Felicia Felix-Mentor, had died and been buried. Twenty-nine years later the dead girl's widower and brother saw her wandering the countryside, dressed in rags, dirty and apparently dumb. She cringed from people as if expecting a beating, and was finally taken into the care of the local hospital, where Zora Hurston went to photograph her. She wrote: 'The sight was dreadful. That blank face with the dead eyes. The eyelids were white all around the eyes as if they had been burned with acid. There was nothing you could say to her or get from her except by looking at her, and the sight of this wreckage was too much to endure for long.'

Was this creature just some imbecile derelict? Or was it really the zombified Felicia Felix-Mentor?

There is no aspect of human life, or death, that Man will not exploit for his own ends. Necromancy is based on the ancient belief that the dead have access to knowledge that is denied to the living. Once across the barrier between life and death our limitations disappear and we are privy to a complete panorama of yesterday, today and tomorrow if, indeed, those concepts continue to have any meaning for us. Necromancers seek to tap that valuable source of information to gain wealth and power, material and intellectual superiority over their fellows, although the few alleged necromancers known to history have not done particularly well out of their grisly pursuit. Edward Kelly, who was the accomplice of Elizabeth I's astrologer, John Dee, died penniless and friendless in the pitch dark of a Dutch jail, with heaven alone knows what foul memories and fears.

Dee himself was said to be successful in raising corpses from their graves to answer his questions and on one occasion, at least, was persuaded to put the pressing query of another to his reanimated cadavers. The matter was urgent: Guy Fawkes wanted to know the outcome of a certain secret project of his. The dead lips uttered 'There will be death', which perhaps should have satisfied Fawkes under the circumstances, but the death proved to be his own and not that of king and parliament as planned.

The seventeenth and eighteenth centuries spawned an hysterical fear of witchcraft and its associated terrors. James I of England, whose obsession with the subject was little short of pathological, passed an anti-witchcraft law that included a clause condemning anyone who might 'take up any dead man, woman or child out of the grave or the skin, bone or any other part of any dead person to be used in any manner of witchcraft, sorcery, charm or enchantment.'

In the occult tradition, adepts in magic must follow age-old rituals to the letter to achieve their aims. The uttering of 'the right words' *must* bring about the realization of their ambitions, though the preparation and training may take a lifetime and take them along paths that may end in their own premature death or madness. But the central premise is if you follow the rules you will always succeed. In necromancy the sorcerer who knows the hideous secret formula can command decaying corpses to assume a semblance of life and bend to his will, like today's alleged zombie masters of Haiti.

Spiritualists, however, describe the loathsome cult of necromancy as *pretended* communication with the dead; for they believe that the dead are beyond the machinations of the living and cannot be forced to do anything against their will. This assumes that the true essence – or personality, or soul, or spirit or whatever one chooses to call it – is actually concerned with the graveyard antics of depraved lunatics.

It is said that Katie King herself chose to materialize, for a limited period only on earth, using the mediumship primarily of Florrie Cook. Carmine Mirabelli, however, was supposed actually to have summoned up the bodily form of a dead poet. In the uneasy world of physical mediumship, where does proof of the survival of death end and necromancy begin?

Even if Katie were genuine, how does her manifestation prove survival? How does the nasty exudation of ectoplasm prove it? Even D.D. Home's spectacular feats show only that he was extraordinarily gifted in highly unusual ways. It was his own interpretation that it was spirit hands that raised him to the ceiling, just as it was God that raised St Teresa and, if it were to happen today, the levitation would probably be ascribed to aliens. Manners maketh man, and fashion maketh phenomena (Chapter 4).

A LITTLE PIECE OF THE MAGIC

With the arrival of the young Israeli Uri Geller on the international scene in the early 1970s, ordinary people – people who believed in anything or people who believed nothing – could capture for themselves a little piece of magic, just by sitting in front of their television sets and watching him bend metal, apparently by the power of his mind alone. And they found they could do the impossible too.

Uri Geller's own career may remain controversial, but his appearance on television sets the world over altered thousands, perhaps millions, of lives forever. Mind over metal is only one highly specialized aspect of psychokinesis (PK) or mind over matter. It may account for a myriad of unexplained phenomena from levitation to raising the dead, for surely a corpse is an inanimate object?

Psychokinesis may be inherent in us all as, to a certain extent, Geller's guruism has shown, but it is strongest when attached to a set of beliefs that *permit* it to happen. One British parapsychologist deliberately, and somewhat cynically, enrolled people for his metal-bending 'classes' from the ranks of the local Spiritualists, because they believed the spirits would help them bend the metal. Their success rate was phenomenally high compared to those coming into the session 'cold'. The impossible is easy to recognize when it is among friends.

Physical mediumship, even if genuine – that is, not fraudulent – can never prove the reality of life beyond the grave, although it may prove many other 'impossibilities' and expose other quaint powers of the human mind and its interaction with the material world. Mental mediumship is altogether easier to come to terms with and is considerably less repulsive to most researchers, to whom ectoplasm is something that should be cured with antibiotics.

A gifted mental medium may be clairvoyant (able to 'see' people and events inaccessible to her through normal means) or clairaudient (able to hear voices and other sounds normally out of the range of our five senses), and convey messages to us that purport to come from deceased friends and relatives. This information is rarely of the dramatic 'don't catch the 11.05 from Euston or else' kind, but often deals with the trivia of our lives such as the colour of the curtains we are *thinking* of buying, or our private worries over a child changing schools.

THE INCREDIBLE IMPORTANCE OF TRIVIA

Sceptics scoff (because they always do, that's their problem), but there is no quicker way to the hardest heart than to have a complete stranger tell you that your dead father 'wants you not to worry about forgetting to post the birthday card to your mother, because she's coming over to see you, and knows you love her anyway'. Mere sentiment, predictable platitudes, might well explain the last part of such a message, but forgetting to send a card is both specific and trivial. It is not the sort of thing a fake medium could find by doing her homework about you in advance, even if she knew exactly who her sitters were going to be. Trivia tells.

The famous British clairaudient Doris Stokes visited the offices of a large London firm in the early 1980s to give a demonstration of her powers to the staff. They had been warned to watch their body language so as not to give Mrs Stokes any hints about who was particularly keen to receive a message from beyond, or to give anything away about themselves. In fact one girl was newly bereaved, her much beloved grannie having died shortly before the visit. This had not been mentioned to Doris, although she could have discovered the fact by shameless homework beforehand.

From what transpired it seems unlikely that she had stooped so low. She not only gave the 'target' hard facts about her life, such as her given name as opposed to the one which she was generally called (something not known to the others in the room), and the health of a distant aunt in the USA (later verified in every detail) but she gave her a personal message purporting to come from the girl's dead child.

The staff grew uneasy – surely June had no child – but Doris was adamant, although very gentle: 'He's yours, love. He *is*. He's grown up over there – he's seven now. He says he forgives you and that you'll know what he means by that.' Tears ran down June's face. She admitted that exactly seven years before she had had an abortion; the child, she had been told, was a boy. Nobody at work knew about that particular part of her past, but somehow Doris had unearthed it. How?

Had the aborted child really 'grown up' in the spirit world, as the Spiritualists believe, and 'come through' to express his forgiveness to his reluctant mother? Or had Doris telepathically picked up June's long-buried trauma that perhaps was crying out to be revealed and forgiven?

Parapsychologists sometimes resort to the theory of 'super-ESP' when faced with such overwhelming evidence for mental mediumship, although they are hard put to explain their explanation. ('It's tapping the collective unconscious...somehow...it's telepathic interaction...er...') It's a lot easier to believe the story as told – that June's dead child had come to Auntie Doris and given her that message – than a complicated network of jargon-filled gobbledygook that leaves you where you started but considerably more confused.

Although the impossible is often apparently without any purpose except mischief, Mrs Stokes' type of cosy familiarity with the sixth sense seems to do some good, to give comfort that can change lives for the better. Katie, if phenomenon she were, was a cosmetic job – art for art's sake. One hopes she did some good for someone, even if it were only William Crookes.

Perhaps the natural talents of psychics like Doris Stokes are beneficent because her Spiritualist beliefs permit her to be open only to healthy and comforting influences. The framework of her philosophy in effect limits her to one type of communication with the impossible. But outside the Spiritualists' slippers-by-the-fire cosiness, the powers of destruction rage unchecked and unpredictable.

3

□ HOLY SMOKE! □

Mrs Carpenter surfaced from her dreams to the troubling smell of burning. The water pump in the garage had been malfunctioning recently, so she got up, went out to turn it off and went back to bed. This was at 5 a.m. on 2 July 1951 in St Petersburg, Florida.

At 8 a.m. Mrs Carpenter was interrupted again, this time by a telegraph boy with a telegram for her tenant, Mrs Mary Reeser. There was something very strange about Mrs Reeser's apartment. As Mrs Carpenter reached the door a wave of heat struck her in the face and the doorknob was too hot to handle. She screamed for help.

With the assistance of two workmen, she entered the apartment. At first it seemed that Mrs Reeser was not there. The superheated air hung thick and heavy, with nothing to account for it; no cooker or heater was on, but curiously there was a small flame dancing over the partition between the gallery kitchen and the living area. Mrs Reeser's bed had not been slept in so they assumed that she had left the flat the night before. But when the authorities were called in to deal with the effects of the heat – presumed fire – they discovered that Mrs Reeser, or rather what was left of her, was still in the apartment. As the official report read:

> Within a blackened circle about four feet in diameter were a number of coiled seat-springs and the remains of a human body.

> Within the remains consisted of a charred liver attached to a piece of backbone a skull shrunk to the size of a baseball, a foot encased in a black satin slipper but burned down to just above the ankle, and a small pile of blackened ashes.

The 'overstuffed easy chair' in which she had been sitting when overcome by this terrifying and inexplicable doom, had been burned down to its springs, but apart from that one small flame on the joist *there was no other evidence of fire in the apartment*. Whatever had consumed Mrs Reeser so utterly had been contained within the cursed 'blackened circle', as if the legendary 'pillar of fire' had materialized in the apartment and brought about her destruction. She had died from spontaneous human combustion (SHC).

Four feet (120 cm) from the ground, as if an invisible plimsoll line had been drawn, the evidence of heat began. The wall was disfigured with smoke, electric fittings were melted or distorted, and an electric clock had been stopped (at 4.20) but curiously, was not broken. It worked when plugged in elsewhere.

The local police were grateful that Dr Wilton Krogman, a forensic fire-death specialist, happened to be in the area, but even he expressed astonishment at the nature of Mrs Reeser's death:

> I cannot conceive of such complete cremation without more burning of the apartment itself. In fact the apartment and everything in it should have been consumed. Never have I seen a human skull shrunk by intense heat. The opposite has always been true; the skulls have either abnormally swollen or have virtually exploded into hundreds of pieces...I regard it as the most amazing thing I have ever seen. As I review it, the short hairs on my neck bristle with vague fear. Were I living in the Middle Ages, I'd mutter something about black magic.

But this was 1951 and the death of the sixty-seven-year-old widow had to be accounted for somehow, preferably with an explanation – that may be improbable but could not be allowed to be impossible.

In this case the public joined in the hunt for The Answer with gusto. Perhaps she had committed a horrible suicide by throwing petrol over herself and igniting it? Perhaps her enemies (she lived quietly and was not known to have any) napalmed her? One correspondent proffered the idea that she had fallen victim to an 'atomic pill', although he was vague as to its nature.

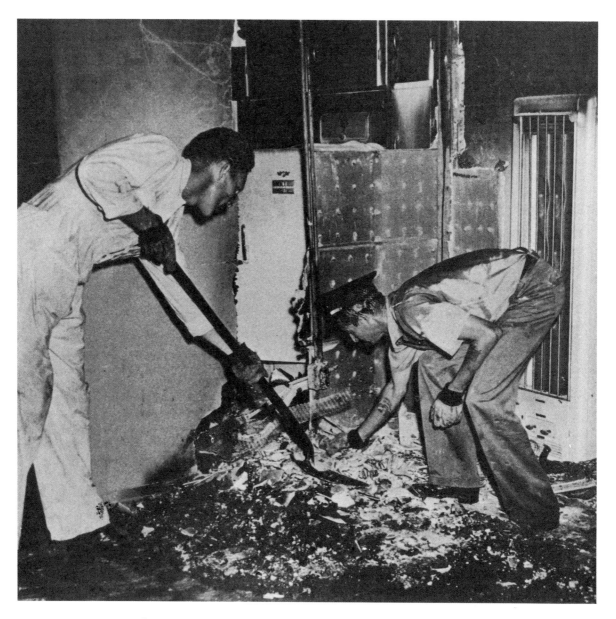

Raking over the remains of Mrs Reeser, whose body was reduced to a sticky liquid by spontaneous human combustion (SHC) on the night of 2 July 1951. Officially, of course, there is no such phenomenon.

An anonymous contributor to the think-tank wrote of having seen a 'ball of fire' in the neighbourhood of Mrs Reeser's flat the night before her death. The FBI were called in, which adds a more sinister note to the proceedings (but unfortunately for the conspiracy theorists the CIA stayed away). Krogman finally reached a conclusion: the victim had been taken elsewhere and done to death by person or persons unknown, and her body had been consumed by some kind of sophisticated mega-heating equipment – except for the grisly bits and pieces that were found. These were taken back to her flat and the murderer(s) made the whole thing look like...whatever it did look like, by themselves melting the electric fittings and stopping the clock. Cleverly, they thought to heat up the doorknob, too.

Even in the face of such expert testimony the police showed unusual reluctance to toe the party line, and at least a year after the discovery of Mrs Reeser's shrunken skull the case was still open.

WHEN THE TRUTH REALLY HURTS

Charles Fort, the American pioneer collector of anomalous phenomena, remarked 'There was never an explanation which did not need an explanation itself.' If Krogman's extraordinary theory were correct, then why didn't the criminals simply burn down the apartment – as many a murderer has done before and since, to cover up the crime? And who owns the sort of equipment necessary to reduce a human being to such a shadow of its former self? Who, besides fictional master-criminals and mad scientists in James Bond movies, would know how to shrink skulls with heat, and bother to heat up the odd doorknob?

The 'authorities' may look the other way when the Cosmic Joker plays most of his tricks, but death by some unexplained fire must be dealt with head on. Because spontaneous human combustion is a fact against nature (as most people understand it) coroners tend to look for an acceptable explanation even if it means avoiding the actual facts like the plague.

Consider the case of the Dewar sisters, Margaret and Wilhemina, both retired school-teachers who lived at Whitley Bay, Northumberland. Margaret, returning home on the evening of 22 March 1908, received no answer when she called out for her sister. Going upstairs she found Wilhemina lying dead of atrocious burns – on an unsinged bed. There was no evidence of fire or even excessive heat in the house. Almost mad with horror, Margaret reported this incredible event to the local police, and then began the shameless hounding of this impeccable witness.

What she had claimed to see was clearly impossible, so she must be lying. Doggedly Margaret stuck to her story, but the coroner reminded her repeatedly that she was giving evidence under oath and perjury was a serious affair. He even adjourned the inquest to give the bereaved woman time to rethink her testimony, but not before allowing a young policeman to swear that she had been so drunk on the night of the death that she had been rambling. He did not reveal how he could distinguish apparent intoxication from abject terror.

During the adjournment intense pressure was put on Margaret – this respectable, abstemious, retired schoolteacher. The neighbours now believed her to be a liar and a drunk and, who knows, possibly a murderess as well. When the inquest recommenced Margaret shakily 'confessed' to having found her badly burned sister *downstairs*, and that she had carried her upstairs, where she died. This, of course, is no more of an 'explanation' than the truth, for how she had been consumed remained a mystery. But downstairs implies a kitchen, and possible sources of fire, so the jury was satisfied. Nothing had been explained; Margaret Dewar had lost her sister and her reputation, and she had looked on hell.

If the facts don't fit then change them;
if the witnesses are obdurate discredit
or destroy them.

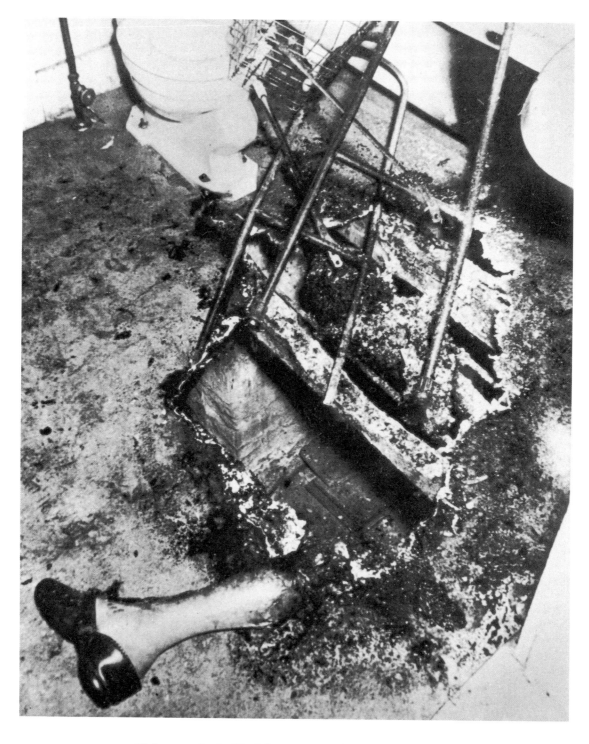

All that remained of Dr John Irving Bentley, a victim of SHC on 5
December 1966. Typically, one portion of limb escapes unscathed, as does
the surrounding furniture. No one knows how or why.

Of all deaths by fire, SHC leaves the most distinctive telltale signs – like a sick, idiosyncratic flourish to round off the horror nicely. A bit of the victim, usually one of the extremities, escapes whole while the rest of the body is reduced to a heap of repulsive soot, or a loathsome sticky liquid. Very little of the surroundings is even scorched, although experts have estimated that to reduce a body to a *liquid* form, heat exceeding 3000°F (1648°C) would be needed. Bodies in crematorium furnaces take hours just for the flesh to burn away even at 2000°F (1093°C), and of course the coffins burn first...

ON THE COSMIC HITLIST

Mrs Sam Satlow of Hoquiam, Oregon died on 7 December 1973 and lay in her coffin in the Chapel of Rest in Coleman's mortuary for three days, with the coffin lid firmly screwed down. In the early hours of 10 December local residents smelled burning and raised the alarm. Police Chief Richard Barnes said 'She was completely consumed to the hips. We have no proof that a crime was committed and no evidence of it...we have no evidence, either, which would point to arson; investigators can't determine the cause...the burning of a woman's body in a coffin inside a locked funeral home remains a mystery.'

She was consumed to the hips, the coffin was merely charred. The extraordinary selectivity of the fire in these cases is one of its most impossible features.

The best 'joke' is to burn someone to a crisp in close proximity to highly inflammable substances, which are left untouched. On Sunday 13 December 1959 in Detroit, Michigan, a motorist saw smoke coming from a wayside garage. Inside was a car that contained a grisly sight. Billy Thomas Peterson was sitting on the driver's seat: 'His left arm was so badly burned that the skin rolled off. His genitals had been charred to a crisp. His nose, mouth and ears were burned...the hairs on his body, his eyebrows, and the top of his head were all unsinged. Even through burned flesh hairs protruded unharmed.' He was still alive, but died shortly after he was discovered.

Billy's jeans and underclothes showed only the slightest signs of heat damage yet a plastic religious statue on the dashboard had melted with the heat. A full tank of petrol had not been touched by the ravages of such appalling fire and there was no sign of fire or heat elsewhere in the garage. Only Billy, part of his seat and a plastic stick-on statuette had suffered from the mysterious and awful fate of spontaneous human combustion.

In this case, the authorities had a ready-made, if entirely implausible, explanation to hand. Billy had been attempting to commit suicide by coupling a pipe to the exhaust of the car and sitting in the driver's seat waiting for a peaceful death to overtake him. This was not to be. But 'obviously' the carbon monoxide fumes had set fire to him...

At least one other would-be suicide is known to have been 'zapped' by the finger of fire that seems to choose its victims according to some cosmic hit list. On 18 September 1952 in Louisiana a Mrs Cousins saw smoke coming from the flat above and rang the fire station. The fireman broke down the door of Mr Glen B. Denney's flat. In the bedroom 'the man was lying on the floor behind the door, and he was a mass of flames. Not another blessed thing in the room was burning...I don't know what caused the fire to burn so hot. He could have been saturated with some oil. I did not smell anything, however. In all my experience, I never saw anything to beat this.'

Mr Denney had been alive when the fire took him, but had attempted to cut his wrists in the *kitchen* – there was blood on the kitchen floor and the body, damaged though it was, revealed the act. Although there were no cans of kerosene, empty or full and no matches around, the coroner decided that the hapless Denney had slit his arteries and then – despite the immediate trauma of spouting arteries –

had walked into the bedroom, poured the phantom kerosene over himself and made himself into a bonfire. Remember there was no smell of oil. The difficulties involved in striking a match with fingers soaked in kerosene and with your lifeblood pumping out in huge gouts are beyond comprehension. But the fact remains that Denney was attempting suicide when he was chosen by fate, God, the Cosmic Joker, what you will – but most improbably by accident – to be consumed by the strangest fire.

Some Christians believe that the mysterious 'sin against the Holy Ghost' for which there is no forgiveness, is suicide. The God of the Old Testament, if not the New, was much given to sending thunderbolts or pillars of fire to destroy the enemies of His Chosen. He rained brimstone and fire upon the cities of the plain, Sodom and Gomorrah 'and lo, the smoke of the country went up as the smoke of a furnace' (Genesis 19). 'By the blast of God they perish, and by the breath of his nostrils they are consumed,' the author of The Book of Job states unequivocally. A burning bush was arranged to catch Moses' attention, and Shadrach, Mesach and Abed-Nego, who were favourites of the Lord, were saved from the super-heated fiery furnace by a mysterious 'Son of God' who appeared in their midst – even their clothes were untouched by the fire and heat. This story admittedly figures in the Book of Daniel, which is widely regarded as a parable and not historical, but it suggests a certain knowledge of how God behaves when angry. The goodies of *Star Wars* uttered their 'May the Force be with You' and felt quite free to zap the opposing forces with laser guns in much the same sort of way.

But not all suicides are pre-empted by paranormal roasting, and even wickedness on a grand scale often fails to raise a flicker of godly fire, at least in this life. Even Hitler's body was consumed by unsatisfactory normal combustion, and that only after he shot himself. If the victims of SHC are indeed selected by some being or committee unknown, then we don't know why. All we do know with any certainty is that the phenomenon exists.

THE FINAL BURNING RAGE

Those who believe in reincarnation see our present existence as a single link in a long and well-forged chain, reaching far into the past and set to reach far into the future. Each life has a specific purpose and carries with it the penalties and rewards incurred through choices made in past existences, when our intrinsic self was masked in a variety of personalities. This 'eye for an eye' type of justice may be spread over many lifetimes but there is no escaping it; karma will get us in the end. Perhaps SHC is a somewhat drastic means of evening up the score.

Nobody enjoys being burnt, but some people do commit suicide by pouring petrol over themselves and setting it alight; it was almost fashionable among Buddhist monks during the 1970s as a protest against war in the world. But that was their final blaze of glory; a life of total passivity had led up to it, and unimaginable discipline permitted them to commit their last act. But there are other forms of suicide, no less an act of will, but unconscious and cumulative. Drug addiction and alcoholism could be said to be forms of creeping suicide; for despair and depression seek oblivion. Most victims of SHC are lonely, possibly suicidal, probably depressed and quite likely repressed. If the halo of the saints can be taken literally, as an outward and visible sign of their inward state of grace, then the sudden fiery deaths of certain individuals could equally represent the burning rage within, the spectacular antithesis to the slow decline of depression, the actual moment of their suicide.

The German psychoanalyst Georg Groddeck proposed that we often externalize our fears and repressions by turning well-known phrases or sayings into psychosomatic illnesses. Thus 'I can't go on any longer' might become an hysterical paralysis, 'I can't face it', becomes blindness and 'I can't put my foot down' literally that. Similarly, doubt about our next step might make us actually slip and fall; taken to extremes this might explain why some go to the blazes in an outburst of fiery rage.

The Roman Catholic Church considers despair to be a sin; perhaps that concept embodies both the psychological and psychic elements that seem to be present in SHC. However, because the fire comes out of the blue and consumes whom it may without warning, we will never know for certain what mental or karmic imbalance invites it to strike.

Of course here we are considering a phenomenon that is definitely impossible. SHC is not a verdict coroners find attractive; it makes them look as if they don't know what they're doing, as if they've lost control. Experts, like the forensic scientist Professor Keith Simpson, do not attempt to explain the unexplainable but prefer, if pressed, to theorize in general about this macabre phenomenon. 'I have not seen a case, in forty years' practice, where I have been satisfied that the body burning is literally spontaneous.' Professor Simpson wrote to Michael Harrison, author of *Fire from Heaven* (1976). Simpson did admit: 'though body fat when deteriorating and oily can burn, some other condition has to be present to start fire...' Because science does not allow for external agencies such as God or E.T., and shakes its head at the notion of psychokinetic power, then deaths by SHC must remain categorized as 'unusual fire deaths'.

THE ONES THAT GOT AWAY

In the 1940s a woman was found, terribly burned on her back in an unscorched bed. She was in such pain that the doctor had to anaesthetize her before dressing the wound. In her few moments of lucidity she said she had 'no idea' how this dreadful thing had happened. She died in hospital very soon afterwards.

There have, however, been survivors of the fire. In 1974 an American, Jack Angel, had his right arm burnt off by a fire that was proved to have started *from within*, but he lived. The source of the fire and the reason for it remains a mystery. Late on the night of 25 May 1985, as reported in the London *Evening Standard*, the *National Enquirer* and *Fortean Times*, 19-year-old Paul Hayes was walking along a road

in Stepney Green, in the East End of London. Suddenly he burst into flames and yet he lived to tell the story:

It was indescribable...like being plunged into the heat of a furnace...My arms felt as though they were being prodded by red-hot pokers, from my shoulders to my wrists. My cheeks were red-hot, my ears were numb. My chest felt like boiling water had been poured over it. I thought I could hear my brains bubbling...I tried to run, stupidly thinking I could race ahead of the flames...I thought I was dying. Images of my parents, my friends, my girlfriend, came to mind...

Then, abruptly, it was over. The flames had vanished and 'there was no smoke'. Shock set in; shivering he staggered to the London Hospital, which was not far away. He was 'numb in some spots and white-hot in others'. He was treated for severe burns. Yet the shirt he was wearing, although bearing extensive scorch marks, had not been consumed in the fire.

One of the most detailed accounts of surviving the fire attack comes from Professor James Hamilton of the Department of Mathematics, the University of Nashville, Tennessee. One freezing evening in January 1805 he was walking home from the campus when he felt 'a steady pain like a hornet sting, accompanied by a sensation of heat' in his left calf. To his astonishment, a blue flame about 15 cm (6 in) long was shooting out of his leg 'about the size of a dime in diameter, and somewhat flattened at the top'. Instinctively, he clapped his hand on to it but it persisted in its offence against nature. So, being a man of education, he decided to stifle it by cupping his hand over the flame thus cutting off the oxygen supply. It went out, never to reappear. Fortunately for the intelligent Professor Hamilton he had not obeyed another basic instinct when faced with fire; he had not tried to douse it with water. Researchers into SHC have discovered this to be a terrible mistake; water makes it worse. This is Alice-land with an X certificate.

The indomitable chronicler of such bizarre incidents, Vincent Gaddis, goes on to describe the aftermath of this extraordinary attempt to burn up the good professor, in his *Mysterious Fires and Lights* (1967):

> On the surface of the outer and upper part of his leg was an injury that resembled an abrasion, about three-fourths of an inch in length, very livid in appearance. It extended from the femoral end of the fibula in an oblique direction towards the upper portion of the gastrocnemii muscles. The wound was extremely dry, and the scar tissue had gathered in a roll at the lower edge of the abraded surface.

The wound took far longer to heal than most burns, and Professor Hamilton's clothing showed the typically 'impossible' signs of damage, suggesting it was no ordinary flame. Although his thick winter underpants revealed a tiny hole, the trousers – despite the fact that the flame had shot through them – bore no sign whatsoever of the event. An ochre-coloured deposit of some kind was found on the inside of the trouser leg, but it was easily scraped off.

The fact that there are survivors seems to indicate that all is not well with the Divine Judgement theory, or the idea that SHC is the sudden retribution for sins committed in this or past lives. If it is merely a warning of some kind, surely it would help if the victims knew precisely what sins they had committed in order to repent, and avoid the fire next time.

ALCOHOL – THE ULTIMATE WARNING

When dealing with the impossible it is perhaps a mistake to assume that there are consistent reasons for any particular type of phenomenon. Are there, for example, meaningful links, common factors among the circumstances or the characters of the victims of SHC? It has been suggested that they are mainly 'elderly females of corpulent habit, addicted to drink' and that they 'all led an idle life.' But Billy

Peterson was not female and Professor Hamilton was neither female nor an idler, but then the attack misfired in his case. Admittedly, Wilhemina Dewar had retired from teaching and could therefore be considered to be 'idle', but she was well-known for her abstemiousness. Yet alcohol, in one form or another, does figure in some of the classic cases of SHC but not, as far as one can tell, because of its intrinsically inflammable properties, but rather as a predisposing factor in the psychic requirements of the phenomenon. Consider the following:

On 19 February 1888 the calcined remains of an anonymous 'old soldier' were found in extraordinary circumstances in a loft in Constitution Street, Aberdeen. Just recognizable, the body lay on a beam, the floor immediately beneath him having burned away. The roof was slightly damaged by the mysterious heat, but only in the strictly localized area above the corpse. Surrounding the dreadful remains were bales of hay, entire and unsinged. The man was a well-known drunk and had been seen going into the loft with a bottle in one hand and a lamp in the other the night before. Witnesses agreed, however, that they had noticed the lamp go out quietly and there had been no fire immediately afterwards. But the 'obvious' case was quickly seized upon – alcoholics and naked flames mean trouble...

At 2.30 one Tuesday morning in 1725 the notorious drunk, Madame Nicolet Millet, was found dead and burning in an unburnt armchair in the hall of her husband's inn in Rheims. It was rumoured that Jean Millet was enamoured of a serving maid and wanted Nicole out of the way. The police promptly arrested him for the callous murder of his wife, but neat though his solution was, they were immediately stymied by the presence of a medical student called Claude-Nicholas Le Cat who was well-read in accounts of SHC. He insisted on an impromptu cross-questioning of the wretched Millet, making it his first priority to establish that the dead woman had been addicted to drink. But he hastened to point out the facts of the case:

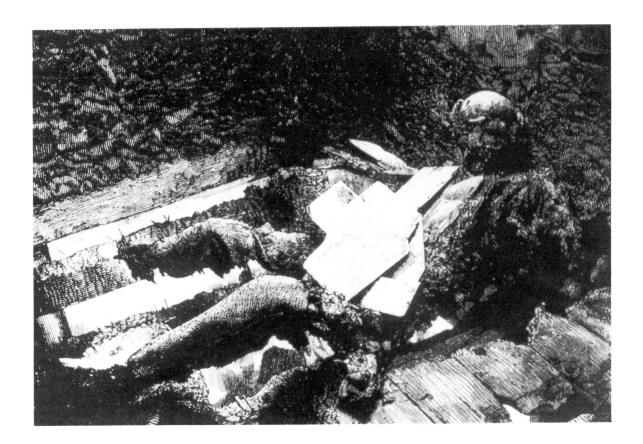

When this old soldier went up in flames on 19 February 1888 in a
Scottish loft, his fondness for alcohol was blamed. Yet no known fire
selects its victim and ignores highly flammable bales of hay...

...pray ask yourself by what human agency such total combustion might be effected? ...Observe how, despite the almost total destruction of the body, the chair in which the dead woman was sitting is hardly burned. True, the leather is somewhat scorched, the varnish of the woodwork somewhat bubbled ...but how could a fire procured by ordinary criminal intent have managed to burn the body in its entirety, whilst leaving unharmed the chair in which the poor woman was sitting?

Ah, said the police (no doubt raising their eyes to heaven, which might have, had they waited, thrown some light on the matter). The husband threw a bottle of brandy over her and set her alight. She fell back on the chair only when the damage to her body had been done, hence the unburnt furniture.

Millet was condemned to face Madame la Guillotine, while Le Cat feverishly consulted his records, comparing this case to other accounts of SHC. He was so persuasive that Millet was acquitted at the eleventh hour. Le Cat's final pronouncement on the case was that Nicole Millet had died 'by visitation of God' due to her intemperate habits. It was, in effect, retribution without warning; instant karma.

A lady given to immersing herself in alcohol, but only as a brisk body-rub, was the unfortunate Countess Cornelia Zangari and

Bandi of Verona. In early April 1731 her maid went to wake her and was hit by a nauseating wave of fetid air, speckled with a sticky soot. As the *Gentlemen's Magazine* for that quarter reported: 'The floor of the chamber was thick-smear'd with a gluish moisture, not easily got off...and from the lower part of the window trickl'd down a greasy, loathsome, yellowish liquor with an unusual stink.'

This was disturbing enough, but a few feet from the undamaged bed was 'a heap of ashes, two legs untouch'd, stockings on, between which lay the head, the brains, half of the back part of the skull and the whole chin burn'd to ashes, among which were found three fingers blacken'd. All the rest was ashes which had this quality, that they left in the hand a greasy and stinking moisture.'

Two candlesticks were among the bulk of undamaged furniture in the room and even the cotton wicks of the candles remained untouched by the fire that had liquidized the Countess. The Scottish scientist Sir David Brewster gave a full account of the incident in his *Letters on Natural Magic* (1842), remarking:

> For an examination of all the circumstances of the case, it has been generally supposed that an internal combustion had taken place; that the lady had risen from her bed to cool herself, and that, on her way to open the window, the combustion had overpowered her, and consumed her body in a process in which no flame was produced which could set fire to the furniture or floor...the Countess Zangari was in the habit, when she felt herself indisposed, of washing all her body with camphorated spirit of wine.

Even among the relatively few people who believed in the phenomenon of SHC, it was commonly held until very recently that alcohol was not merely a predisposing factor in causing the fire, but the one and only cause.

This too, too, neat theory brought together a physical explanation, albeit fallacious (alcoholics are naturally highly inflammable) with a moral one (God is not mocked).

But even human beings whose veins would seem to run with Polish vodka are still basically bags of water. Experiments with oil-soaked human fat indicate the impossibility of maintaining the sort of flame that burns so thoroughly that it consumes the flesh utterly and of creating any kind of fire that selects flesh and ignores furniture or clothing.

DO MURDERERS READ DICKENS?

Charles Dickens, in his horrifying description of Krook's death by SHC in *Bleak House*, draws a moral: 'Call the death by any name...attribute it to whom you will, it is the same death eternally – inborn, inbred, engendered in the corrupt humours of the vicious body itself, and that only – Spontaneous Combustion, and none other of all the deaths that can be died.'

This is the only account of SHC ever encountered by most people, and horrifying though it is, remains for them pure, whimsical fiction. But Dickens was familiar with real-life cases, and he certainly believed in SHC. No doubt he would have been fascinated to know that Dr Wilton Krogman, in his investigation of the destruction of Mrs Reeser (p 57) was, according to *Today* magazine: '... impressed by the almost uncanny resemblance to the *Bleak House* episode. His suspicion is that the murderer was someone who knew a lot about burning, and who read a lot of Dickens ' — a novel variation on the 'copy-cat' murder theme.

It is worth looking at Dickens' skilful and theatrical use of symbolism in the scene where William Guppy and Tony Weevle discover the truth about Krook's death. They enter the grim house in the squalid alley with more than their usual trepidation: 'What's the matter with the cat?' says Mr Guppy. 'Look at her!' 'Mad, I think. And no wonder, in this evil place.'

Countess Zingari's lap dog was found cowering with terror in the outer chamber, driven mad by the stinking liquid ooze that had once been its mistress. Here it is a cat, traditionally associated with dark forces, that has

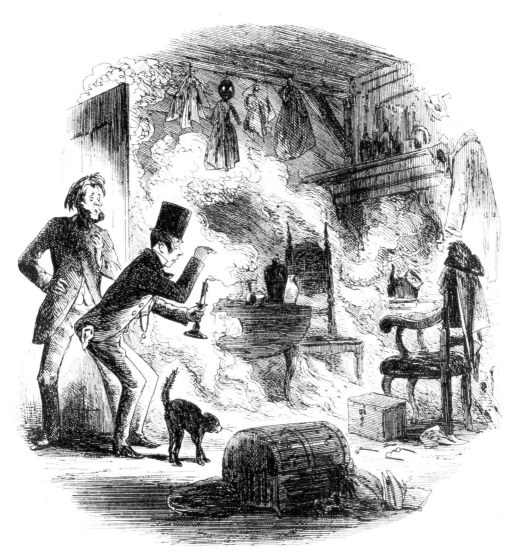

suffered as witness to the holocaust. (Perhaps Dickens was subconsciously evoking Le Cat, the medical student who figured so significantly in the Millet case.)

As the two men reluctantly penetrate the inner rooms, the cat slinks to the doorway of the back shop and:

When Dickens killed off Krook by SHC in *Bleak House* readers commonly supposed the phenomenon to be the result of the author's over-heated imagination. Yet Dickens was familiar with well-documented cases of this weird and appalling death, and believed it to be a real, if rare, occurrence, triggered by the moral decay of the victim.

stands snarling – not at them; at something on the ground, before the fire...there is a smouldering suffocating vapour in the room, and a dark greasy coating on the walls and ceiling. The chairs and table, and the bottle so rarely absent from the table, all stand as usual...the cat remains...still snarling at something on the ground...What is it? Hold up the light.

Here is a small burnt patch of flooring; here is the tinder from a little bundle of burnt paper, but not so light as usual, seeming to be steeped in something; and here is – not the cinder of a small charred and broken log of wood sprinkled with white ashes, or is it coal? O Horror, he IS here! and this from which we run away, striking out the light and overturning one another into the street...

Generations of readers have boggled at this scene, as well they might, and countless reams of examination paper have been filled with criticism of the master story-teller for his 'excessive symbolism that loses the reader because it loses credibility'... (the author quotes, with shame, from her own Eng. Lit. finals). Dickens made Krook die from SHC that was triggered by festering moral decay. He could find no harsher judgement for him. But the grisly scene was drawn, in detail, from life – from fact, not fiction.

THE CINDERS SYNDROME

It seems as if most victims of SHC die alone, but there have been witnesses to the abrupt visit-ation of flame. On 27 August 1938 twenty-two-year-old Phyllis Newcombe was dancing with her fiancé Henry McAusland at the Shire Hall 'hop', Romford, Essex. At the end of the dance she was suddenly enveloped in blue flame, which McAusland tried to beat out with his hands, but 'within minutes' she had turned into 'a blackened mass of ash'. The crinoline-style frock she was wearing was blamed at the inquest for being intrinsically inflammable (precise reasons not stated), and the inevitable accidental brush with a lighted match or cigarette evoked. The dead girl's father, how-ever, produced a piece of material that had been used to make the ball gown and deliber-ately applied a lighted cigarette to it. It would not burn. The coroner admitted: 'In all my experience I have never come across a case as mysterious as this.'

Another sick variation on the line: 'You shall go to the ball, Cinders', was the horren-dous case of nineteen-year-old Maybelle Andrews who was dancing with her boyfriend Billy Clifford in a nightclub in London's Soho in the 1920s. Flames suddenly burst from her back, setting fire to her hair. A badly shaken Clifford, who was himself burnt by trying to beat out the flames, said afterwards that they seemed to come *from within* the victim, who died in the ambulance.

One of the most recent, and most con-fused, cases of apparent SHC was that of Jackie Fitzsimon, a cookery student at Halton College of Further Education, Widnes in Cheshire, who burst into flames on 28 January 1985. She was walking down the corridor with some friends five minutes after the end of a cookery examination and suddenly felt intense heat on her back. Within seconds she was on fire and died fifteen days later in 'intensive care'. The story was seized by the media, at first locally and then nationally, as a clear case of SHC, thus ensuring that it would be the last verdict even the most broad-minded coroner would advise the jury to bring in, even if it meant ignoring the facts totally. This is what happened.

The 'obvious' explanation was that her cookery smock had caught fire and had smoul-dered unnoticed for a few minutes before ignit-ing the girl's back. As far as the Coroner was concerned, the cookery connection was a god-send. With typical selectivity he heard evidence only from the witnesses who were likely to uphold the acceptable verdict of 'misadven-ture'.

The Cheshire Fire Brigade had called in investigations from the Shirley Institute at Manchester (who were responsible for the tests into the Boeing 737 disaster at Manchester air-port in August 1985). These two expert bodies compiled a thirty-page report on Jackie's death, which proved to their satisfaction that her clothes could not have caught fire from an accidental brush with the cooker five minutes before. The coroner decided not to use the document as evidence. Moreover, not a single representative of the Fire Brigade was called as a witness.

The Home Office chemist, Philip Jones, proved that a similar cookery jacket could smoulder for a maximum of thirty seconds before the fumes would be noticed. Jackie's smock went up in flames *five minutes* after she left the alleged source of heat, the cooker. And the nearest she could have been to a burner was 20 cm (8 in) away.

One of the students who witnessed the

tragedy, spoke of a cigarette falling down Jackie's back, but later amended this to 'a strange glowing light' above Jackie's right shoulder. Whatever it was, the poor girl had screamed: 'It's gone down my back – get it out!' which certainly points to a tangible object, such as a cigarette, being the culprit. At the time, probably due to shock, Jackie seemed strangely free from pain. She was rushed to hospital, where she was discovered to have suffered 13% burns 'on her buttocks and back from bra to pantie line' – hardly severe enough to have caused her death. In fact, when the police interviewed her at the hospital (*two days* after the incident) she was happily sitting up and chatting. Two weeks later she died of 'shock-lung' by which time the CID had been called in (as were the FBI in the case of Mrs Reeser's death) and the witnesses seemed to have become hopelessly confused between what really happened and the pressure to come up with an acceptable explanation.

The British journal of anomalous phenomena, the *Fortean Times* (named after Charles Fort) issue 47, carried the report of the Fitzsimon inquest by authors Peter A. Hough and Jenny Randles, who had been invited to attend it by the police. They said: 'We were expecting great things – after all, the official enquiry had lasted several months, and had involved fire officers and other governmental and police departments – but we saw no scientific and polished presentation of the facts. Instead we were offered a barrage of weak sloppy investigation and amazing cop-outs.'

The coroner had begun the proceedings 'by advising the jury to ignore all the talk in the media about SHC'. The 'impossible' out of the way, they chose to fashion an acceptable verdict out of the improbable, espousing the cooker-flame theory, one that was disproved several times by the experts. (A phantom cigarette would have confused matters further by implicating one of the other students and there was no evidence that any of them had been smoking.)

But why did the coroner suppress the thirty-page report by the fire experts? Why did the police request the presence at the inquest of two well-known writers on anomalous phenomena? Why did Jackie die with only superficial burns, when she had appeared to be so well shortly after the 'accident'? Why were the CID called in? Why had it taken two days for the uniformed branch to bother to investigate the incident?

The media, who had been uncharacteristically eager to espouse the SHC explanation, fell completely for the coroner's verdict: 'Rumours that cookery student Jacqueline Fitzsimon ... died of spontaneous human combustion were not true, it emerged from an inquest last week', the local paper stated flatly.

It would be a most unusual inquest that returned a verdict of death by SHC. Most coroners, as we have seen, agree with Dr Gavin Thurston, the coroner for West London, who has stated: 'no such phenomenon as spontaneous combustion exists, or has ever occurred.' But there is at least one exception that proves the rule: on 3 April 1970 an inquest was held into the death of eighty-nine-year-old Mrs Margaret Hogan of Prussia Street, Dublin. The City Coroner, Dr P. J. Bofin, stated (as reported in the *Irish Times* of 12 May):

> There is no doubt that the woman died from burning [she was, in fact, reduced to 'a mere pile of ashes']. The circumstances of the burning are unusual, and would conform to what is called Spontaneous Combustion. Spontaneous Combustion does not mean that the fires are in fact spontaneous in origin. It's simply a term carried on in forensic literature to describe a set of circumstances in which a person is burned to death without an obvious source of fire...

It would be interesting to know which 'forensic literature' acknowledges SHC in so many words, although Michael Harrison in *Fire From Heaven* claims to have seen 'the entry "Spontaneous Combustion" again and again under the heading "suspected cause of fire", in the report-sheets of the London Fire Brigade...' But the Press Officers deny all knowledge of such entries.

Ironically, in the case of Jackie Fitzsimon the media's initial sensational reporting of apparent SHC did more harm than good, making the coroner more obdurate in seeking a normal, rather than a paranormal verdict. The attention-seeking Joker got too much, too late. Or perhaps that was his intention; newspapers will be distinctly unenthusiastic to report cases of SHC now the Fitzsimon case was 'proved' to be plain 'misadventure'. The Joker delights in ruining the reputation of his friends.

But SHC was given its own BBC television coverage on *Newsnight*, (13 January 1986) and in an article that appeared three days later in *The Listener* by the television reporter Steve Bradshaw, who made no bones about the fact that he had set out to discredit a paranormal explanation for a mysterious death by fire. He was to undergo a marked conversion.

On 6 January 1980 the body of seventy-three-year-old Henry Thomas of Ebbw Vale, South Wales, was found in disturbing circumstances and the police were called in. CID officer John Haymer (as reported in *The Listener* and later the *Fortean Times*) described the scene:

> It was a very cold day, but I was struck by the warmth of the house, and the living room was like an oven...the room had a strange glow, orange-red. Condensation was running down the window. The walls were generating heat; the window and the light bulb were covered in an orange substance. The light bulb was bare because the plastic shade had melted. There was an open grate, but it was undisturbed. The settee still had its loose covers. The carpet was largely undamaged. The knobs of the TV had melted, but it was still on.
>
> On the floor was a pair of human feet clothed in socks. They were attached to the lower portion of the body; this was clad in trousers, undamaged as far as a distinct burn-line. From the trousers protruded the calcined bone, and just beyond the knees this disintegrated into an amorphous mass of ash. My first thought was, 'This is just how Dickens described the death of Mr Krook – spontaneous human combustion.'

Fortean Times describe Haymer as a 'well-read Peeler', as indeed he was. But everything about this case accords so precisely with the classic cases of SHC that one is not surprised to find the supporting players apparently reading from some archetypal script. The standard line was also taken by pathologist Professor David Gee in words only too familiar:

> The person collapses and dies for some reason...they fall into the fireplace, or some other form of ignition. Since this usually happens to old ladies, in wintertime, they're probably wearing a lot of clothes. Once the clothing burns, it melts the body fat, which soaks into the clothing...like a candle, with the wick outside. Of course when it gets to the knees, the clothing effectively ends. And that's why the extreme end of the body is rarely damaged.

Strangely enough this highly scientific explanation struck neither the Coroner (who returned an open verdict) nor would-be debunker Bradshaw as fitting the facts of the case. (As Charles Fort wrote: 'A great many scientists are good impressionists: they snub the impertinences of detail.')

The programme took a dramatic U-turn; the manager of a crematorium was asked for his professional comments on pictures of SHC victims. He was frankly perplexed, remarking: 'It looks as if the fire comes from within. Don't ask me how – I've never heard of spontaneous human combustion. But it wants a lot of explaining...and must be frightening.'

Newsnight left the viewer disturbed but comforted with the belief that SHC is a rare phenomenon – after all, the case of Henry Thomas was then six years old. There is no such comfort for us. Even official records show dozens of classic cases, and just how many others are suppressed deliberately by rationalist authorities, ascribed perhaps to 'smoking in bed'? (But did the *bed* smoke?).

Where children are concerned, tragic fires are frequently ascribed to their playing with fire, but Peter Seaton's incineration could hardly fit that theory for he was just eleven months old. One night early in January 1939 the child was put to bed, already half asleep. Shortly afterwards his terrible screams were heard by a visitor, Harold Huxstep, who rushed upstairs and flung open the bedroom door. According to *The Daily Telegraph's* report of the case on 4 January, Mr Huxstep said: 'It seemed as if I had opened the door of a furnace. There was a mass of flames, which shot out, burning my face and flinging me back across the hall. It was humanly impossible to get Peter out.' *The Daily Telegraph* at least was in no doubt about the cause of little Peter's conflagration – spontaneous human combustion.

Little Peter was not an elderly female addicted to drink, and his opportunities for committing sins grievous enough to call down God's fiery wrath had been pathetically limited, in this life anyway.

GREAT BALLS OF FIRE

One of the few tenable theories involving rare but natural causes for SHC first appeared in the international Fortean journal *Pursuit* in 1975, in which Livingstone Gearhart showed the relationship between reported cases of SHC and a rise in solar activity, which affects the earth's magnetic field. A rapid change in the intensity of geomagnetic activity can produce the curious phenomenon of ball lightning, itself until recently outlawed by scientists as impossible, mythological flim-flam. Remember that an anonymous letter told the investigating officers that 'a ball of light' had been seen near Mrs Reeser's apartment the night before her grim remains were found. In *Fate* magazine for May 1961 the Reverend Winogene Savage wrote of an incident where a friend heard his wife scream. She was burning on the floor of the living room, already blackened by the blaze, with a ball of blue fire hovering over her. She and her clothes were destroyed, but nothing in the room was damaged, not even the carpet under her.

Very little is known about the behaviour of ball lightning, although it seems much more common than is generally supposed. A friend of the author tells of standing at her front door one hot, sunny day when to her astonishment, a huge blue ball spitting purplish flares 'a bit like sparklers on bonfire night' rolled straight at her. Terrified she stepped aside; the ball seemed to hesitate 'as if deciding whether to go for me or not' but it rolled past into the house, avoided her petrified brother and went out of the back door, which was fortunately open. Once in the back garden it disintegrated, leaving a pungent smell similar to sulphur, but nowhere was there any trace of burning.

Victims of SHC are roasted from within, as if subjected to a quick burst in a horribly intense microwave oven. In their *Taming of the Thunderbolts* (1969) researchers into ball lightning, Maxwell Cade and Delphine Davis, find that highly specialized circumstances – such as a marked change in the atmospheric conditions – could release enormous amounts of short radio waves in the form of ball lightning. If this happened, it would be 'possible for victims to be burned to death, not merely within their clothes, but even within their skin, either by the proximity of a lightning ball or by having a ball form within their own body...'

But why do some people fall prey to the lightning bolts while most of us (so far) escape being fried?

It seems hard to find a common physiological factor in the deaths of Jackie Fitzsimon, Mrs Reeser, Peter Seaton and Billy Peterson, but what of a psychic trigger? It may be a certain type of fear, residual, perhaps, even in the chatting Jackie after her cookery examination, and implicit in a child like little Peter waking alone, possibly from a nightmare. Or the creeping suicide of despair might alter the body's electromagnetic field, which attracts ball lightning, or even creates it.

Whatever it is, the holocaust breaks out from the very core of our being. The fire could be latent in us all, normally contained by a complex set of variables, a fine balance of the physical, the psychosomatic and the psychic.

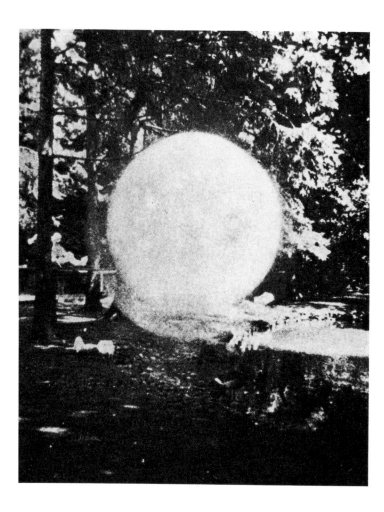

Left A mystery light photographed in the Zoological Gardens in Basle, Switzerland in 1907. Strange lights and fires have been reported throughout history, but only now are scientists taking at least one related phenomenon, ball lightning, seriously. These electrical spheres have been blamed for many unexplained incidents, from the fire of York Minster in 1984 to SHC.

Opposite An artist's impression of a fireball encountered during a storm in Salagnac, France in 1845. It was probably ball lightning.

The human 'aura', so graphically described throughout history by the saintly and the sensitive, may be the gentle glow of the fire within (always with us in life) which, if aggravated according to some cosmic law, causes our death in an explosion of self-destruction.

Charles Fort would possibly disagree. He said: 'I think our data relate not to "spontaneous combustion of human bodies" but to things or beings, that with a flaming process consume men and women, but like werewolves or alleged werewolves, mostly pick women.' He could have been joking, it's often hard to tell with Fort. But if he's right and we are being 'played with' by a capricious cosmic kid then there is a sort of intelligence directing the fire, whither it goes. The tease is that just when one

thinks it safe to point the finger – only suicides, drunks and the desperate get fried – data come along showing that babes and innocently dancing girls are also horribly consumed.

STUCK IN THE COSMIC CHIMNEY

The intelligence could sometimes make a mistake and pick the wrong victims. Perhaps the ancient Greeks were right and the gods are fallible; guilty or innocent, we may simply be in the wrong place at the wrong time.

When I was a child of about eight I had a vision of a woman's head and although she spoke to me, I was too terrified to absorb much of what she said. After a while she grew irri-

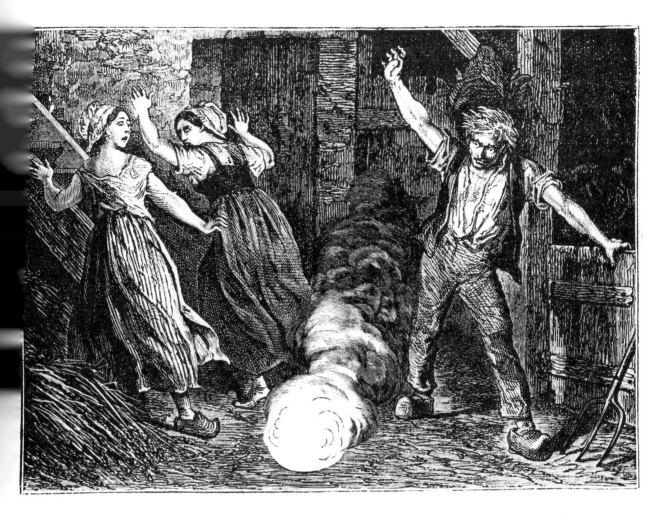

tated with me and seemed to consult other personages beyond the range of my senses. She became angry; it emerged that the vision and the message, so elaborately stage-managed on some other plane, was not meant for me.

Who is to say that the intended victim of the gods was actually living in the next house or the next street to little Peter Seaton but the fire simply missed them and destroyed him instead? Or perhaps the timescale was wrong and the combustion was meant for someone who lived on that spot 100 years ago, or will live there 50 years hence?

Another 'Fortean' theory that is outrageous enough to satisfy friends of the impossible also centres on the concept of a botched attempt by the Joker: what if the charred remains of the victims are the aftermath of a failed 'beam-me-up-Scottie'-type teleportation? Denizens of other worlds may be crying out for sample humans. There are enough unexplained disappearances to account for *successful* experiments in teleportation, after all. Naturally, the aliens, gods, or whoever, would want a cross-section of human life; hence, the baby, the old soldier, the pretty dancing girls, the elderly ladies, the cookery student...And if the victim's resistance is lowered by depression or physical and psychic weakness then so much the easier to snatch them away. Some will inevitably be too weak (or perhaps too strong) for the attempt to be successful and unfortunately they get, as it were, stuck in the cosmic chimney, and are burned to a crisp.

Spontaneous human combustion is so spectacular that it could also be a deliberate decoy, intended to distract us from a wider and even more disturbing attack from beyond. The *Fortean Times* (issue 45) carried a tragic, intriguing tale of a mysterious fire from 1985 under the heading: 'Beware of the Red Monster'. Six-year-old Anthony Raynor of Exeter, Devon, had rushed with terror into his parents' bedroom one night crying: 'A red monster is coming to burn the house down – he's got purple eyes!'

Because of his distress he was taken into his parents' bed; during the night a fire broke out in the children's bedroom. Richard, aged two, and Jason who was four, were rescued but died of burns later. The origin of the fire has not been discovered. Is this story evidence for the existence of Fort's 'things or beings that with a flaming process consume men and women'?

THE INVISIBLE ARSONISTS

Children figure rarely in *known* cases of SHC, but they certainly seem to attract anomalous fires of other sorts, most commonly as part of a poltergeist attack. Indeed, if modern theories about the nature of poltergeists is correct, the apparent victim or focus is actually the culprit, whom, it seems, operates a sort of psychokinetic vandalism through subconscious manipulation.

Outbreaks usually occur in houses where there is a pubescent, or deeply distressed child or teenager. The physical and psychological adjustments involved in growing up, or the flaring up of some resentment or unresolved conflict seems to trigger a spate of frightening phenomena. Lights switch themselves on and off, water drips through ceilings or mysteriously floods empty rooms, rude and sometimes obscene graffiti appears on walls, objects fly unaided through the air and the sound of smashing crockery is reminiscent of a Greek restaurant on New Year's Eve. Then there are the fires. Usually they are small examples of apparently spontaneous combustion in empty rooms, and often they quench themselves before real harm is done.

Although some poltergeist children are boys, most are females undergoing some physiological or psychological crisis. One spectacular series of phenomena was never reported in the media nor investigated by 'ghostbusters'. The story concerns events and people well-known to this author, who has no intention of giving real names, dates or places. (Thus, as 'evidence' it is worthless, the term 'anecdotal' being anathema to scientist and parapsychologist alike. This book is not for them, however.)

The case centred round a teenage girl, who we shall call Julie. She was the adopted daughter of a mentally disturbed woman, 'Mrs Hall', currently going through the menopause. This explosive psychic mixture was exacerbated by their house itself; built by Mrs Hall's late father, it seemed to be steeped in the resentments of their family tensions and tragedies. She had been born in the house. Julie had seen what she later discovered must have been the ghost of her grandfather, wandering about on the upstairs landing looking worried. Visitors grew visibly nervous in such a highly-charged atmosphere and eventually the Hall family were left strictly alone.

The whole thing came to a head for two years in the 1960s, when Julie and her mother engaged in head-on personality clashes. Raps began over Julie's bed, apparently coming from inside the wall, always at 3.30 in the morning. There would be one enormous reverberating rap to wake her up, and as she sat there in the dark terrified and hoping that she had just dreamt it, there came another one, so loud that it shook the bed. Switching on the bedside lamp only added to the nightmare, for the light went on and off, although it remained switched on, and distinct scrabbling noises began to come from the skirting board. There were no mice or other creatures in the house. These phenomena would last for about half an hour at a time while Julie lay awake, petrified with fear. She knew instinctively that there was no point in waking her mother for she was sure that in some inexplicable way, her mother was behind it all.

Soon, however, even the hours of daylight were punctuated by increasingly bizarre happenings; books turned themselves upside down on shelves in empty rooms – sometimes in just a few seconds. After one particularly violent row between Julie and Mrs Hall in which savage remarks were made about Julie's adoption, a book was found lying on her mother's bed. It was *Jane Eyre*, the classic tale of a downtrodden but rebellious little girl, and a favourite of Julie's. On another occasion a copy of *The Heart Has Its Reasons* (by the Duchess of Windsor) hit the girl on the back of the neck as she was crossing the 'haunted' landing. There was no one in the house at the time. Then the fires began.

First there were electrical malfunctions; 'classic' poltergeist manifestations. The television, although switched off and unplugged, suddenly leapt into life showing jagged lines zipping across the screen and accompanied by high-pitched static through which the sound of a woman sobbing could be clearly heard. This happened – and was witnessed by Julie and her father – twice, before the set combusted (during a programme about an abandoned baby). Flames shot up from the back of the set and licked at the curtains, which began to smoulder. Julie jumped up to pull them down while her father unplugged the set, but just as abruptly as it had started the fire stopped. The set was broken but the curtains, which had been well alight, were, somewhat curiously, only frayed. Shaken, they were surveying the damage when they smelled burning coming from the sitting room. Julie's homework was on fire; a school textbook and a half-finished essay on reproduction in mammals was blazing merrily on an occasional table. (Julie wondered grimly whether her science teacher would believe that the homework had suffered spontaneous combustion as the result of a poltergeist attack. On the whole she thought she wouldn't.)

Going upstairs, Julie stumbled on another book that had appeared on the stairs, *The Water Babies*. Some weeks later a box of burnt-out candles was found at the bottom of Julie's wardrobe; although the box itself was charred, none of the clothes hanging next to it had been scorched and no one had smelt burning. All the lightbulbs in the house 'blew' on the same day – the day before Julie's fifteenth birthday – although there was nothing wrong with the wiring, and new light bulbs behaved normally. On her birthday the front door caught fire from inside. The neighbours began to take an interest, especially as they had heard sounds of voices raised in anger and violent sobbing for some weeks. The phenomena were becoming public, but just when they were attracting attention, they stopped.

TRESPASSERS WILL BE...

The Halls' case is particularly interesting, however, because the next family to live in that house suffered from such intense poltergeist attacks that they called in an exorcist. They were the Gattings, a young couple with a baby. Nothing in their lives had prepared them for the barrage of raps on walls, ceilings and windows; heavy footsteps on the stairs and the landing; taps and lights switching themselves on and off, flying crockery, bent cutlery and the front door developing a gaping hole 'as if it had been kicked in from the inside'. The baby screamed almost continuously and then Mrs Gatting developed nervous rashes and suffered blinding headaches. She said: 'We were definitely being forced out by some evil thing, maybe the ghost of somebody who resented us being there. But what decided us to get the priest in was the outbreak of fires. So far it had just been upsetting, but in the end we thought "he" was actually trying to murder us. I didn't relish the idea of being roasted in my bed in that house, so that's when we decided to put a stop to it.'

A cardboard box under their bed began to smoulder in the middle of the night. They put it out with a glass of water, and got up to make a cup of tea only to have the candlewick bedspread go up in flames behind their backs. The child's rattle was found distorted as if it had melted then 'set' again. The smell of burning permeated the entire house continually.

The exorcism worked; all was quiet in that house but even so the Gattings left it forever just six months after they had moved in. There were no further reports of paranormal attack within those walls; perhaps the new owners were made of sterner stuff, or perhaps the 'ghost' had really been sent packing.

Parapsychologists talk of poltergeists being 'place-centred' as in most cases, or 'person-centred', but the phenomena in this case refuse to be so neatly labelled. The Gattings' disturbances seemed to emanate from the house itself, but it was the antagonism of the Hall women who had somehow triggered off the latent paranormal violence in the house. Even at university Julie was visited by raps on her window (four storeys from the ground) – once with such savagery that the glass was cracked. Meanwhile, Mrs Hall reported the strange behaviour of objects that moved around unbidden at her new house. Even today, more than twenty years on, Julie's visits home begin with a spate of self-destructing light bulbs at both her home and her mother's. On two occasions, both the night before a visit, the contents of a plastic waste bin have combusted in unattended rooms in Julie's flat. The correlation between the repressed resentment and the externalized 'flaring up' is obvious, but why did the phenomena increase in severity when the new family moved into the house? Could it really be that the ghost of the grandfather objected to strangers moving into his family home – the house he had built, lived and died in?

Spirits are very, very unfashionable, especially among parapsychologists, who see all poltergeist phenomena as PK (psychokinesis), triggered off by psychological crises. In this case it might be assumed that the Gattings had heard rumours that the house was 'disturbed' and their fear, coupled with the natural problems involved in setting up their first home and bringing up a baby on a limited income, was

itself the signal to bring on the empty horses of the impossible show. It's a theory.

POLTERGEIST-PRONE PEOPLE

Poltergeist children tend to be polite, quiet and well-behaved. They may be the only children in the street who aren't vandals; they often have difficulties expressing emotions or in allowing themselves to acknowledge anger and resentment. Instead of throwing tantrums themselves, they either cause outbreaks of senseless – and often childish – violence through psychokinetic manipulation of their surroundings; or, they invite chaos into their homes by being psychically wide open to the demons of destruction. Some 'victims' of poltergeist attack may be abnormally creative, and the phenomena merely a side effect (albeit excessively theatrical) of the creative process.

The British healer Matthew Manning began his psychic 'career' as a focus for spectacular poltergeist activity, both at his parents' Cambridge home and at boarding school. All the dining room furniture would regularly form itself into complicated heaps when there was no one at home. Strange noises were heard and the classic repertoire of poltergeist's special effects trotted out, even for investigators. But Matthew soon discovered that he could control the phenomena by channelling his psychic and creative energies into some other activity. He began 'automatic drawing' in which drawings and paintings in the style of Beardsley, da Vinci and Monet 'came through' Matthew, and were even graciously signed by them. While he was engaged in this, the poltergeist activity abruptly ceased, but as soon as he took a break from his artistic mediumship, the furniture rebelled once more. Now that he is working full-time on what he considers to be the ultimate form of creativity, healing, he is no longer bothered by anomalous events.

Modern research has shown that the right-hand side of the brain is concerned with creativity, intuition and non-rational thinking, while the left-hand side of the brain copes with logic and analytical ability. In crises, women switch on the right side, relying on a creative or intuitive solution to the problem, while men let the left-hand side come up with a more down-to-earth approach to get them out of trouble. Significantly, more women than men experience all aspects of the paranormal; there are more female mediums than male, traditionally more women than men become witches, girls outnumber boys as poltergeist victims, and more women than men (as far as we know) die by SHC...Is the common link an intense but perverted surge of creativity? Or does the panic implicit in psychological crises cut off the normalizing influence of the left-hand brain, laying women open to the chaotic occult forces inside and outside us all, just waiting to pounce? Perhaps there is something in the ancient idea of 'possession' after all.

ENTER THE INCENDIARY BEING

For friends of the impossible, theories are dangerous. Like explanations, which require explanations, theories are self-indulgent and addictive. They breed in the night and, like the spoilt brats of science, take us over so that we only acknowledge events that fit them, discarding everything else as embarrassingly anomalous. Theories are the missionaries that bring back lost sheep into the fold of the Great Conspiracy. Charles Fort had great fun with theories. In his book *Lo!* he tells of a SHC victim: 'In London, a woman sat asleep, near a grate, and something, as if taking advantage of this means of commonplace explanation, burned her, behind her. Perhaps a being of incendiary appetite had crept up behind her, but I had no data upon which so to speculate...'

But there were data, Fort believed, to substantiate a theory that a *being* had wreaked havoc at Binbrook Farm, Lincolnshire during the winter of 1904–5. Objects were hurled about by unseen hands, 226 out of 250 chickens were mutilated in what seemed to be a ritual manner – the skin of their necks being ripped off, the windpipe pulled out and snap-

ped – and a servant girl burst into flames as she swept the floor. The farmer described the incident to a reporter from the *Louth and North Lincolnshire News*:

> Our servant girl, whom we had taken from the workhouse, and who had neither kin nor friend in the world that she knows of, was sweeping the kitchen. There was a very small fire in the grate: there was a guard there, so that no one can come within two feet or more of the fire, and she was at the other end of the room, and had not been near. I suddenly came into the kitchen, and there she was, sweeping away, while the back of her dress was afire. She looked round, as I shouted, and, seeing the flames, rushed through the door. She tripped, and I smothered the fire out with wet sacks. But she was terribly burned, and she is at Louth Hospital, now, in terrible pain.

The reporter added: 'This last sentence is very true. Yesterday our representative called at the hospital, and was informed that the girl was burned extensively on the back, and lies in a critical condition. She adheres to the belief that she was in the middle of the room, when her clothes ignited.'

Fort noted:

> ...if we accept that, at Binbrook Farm, something was savagely killing chickens, we accept that whatever we mean by a *being* was there. It seems that, in the little time taken by the farmer to put out the fire of the burning girl, she could not have been badly scorched. Then the suggestion is that, unknown to her, something behind her was burning her, and that she was unconscious of her own scorching flesh. All the stories are notable for absence of outcry, or seeming unconsciousness of victims that something was consuming them.

There is something familiar in the story of the serving girl, the girl taken in from the workhouse, without family or a friend in the world, who was sweeping the floor, going round and round, round and round...Where was she in her *mind*? Dancing with Prince Charming, forgetting to keep her eye on the clock? You shall go to the ball, *Cinders*.

THE JOKER'S NAME GAME

This childish 'lexilink' is how the Joker chooses many of his victims. The word-association fiend who occasionally chooses to rule our fates was on particularly good form in June 1986, as this report from *Fortean Times* shows:

> Peter Jones from Bournemouth kept what he thought was a 'lucky' horseshoe charm in his Colt car: he changed his mind after driving past a pub called the Three Horseshoes near Exeter, when the Colt was in collision with three runaway horses. His face was cut when two of the horses tried to jump over his car, smashing the windscreen and onto the roof. The horses were unhurt.

Or, take the case of the seventy-five-year-old spinster, Edith Thompson, found burned up in a charred armchair on 16 February 1972. Apparently she had been dead for two days. There were two 'jokes' involved (possibly more). One: at the time she had been devoured by SHC she had 'apparently been lighting a fire' but, as Michael Harrison points out, she had not succeeded in doing so. Secondly, it happened fifty years after another Edith Thompson (and her lover Frederick Bywaters), had been hanged for murdering her husband. The Edith Thompson who was to end her long and lonely life in a ball of flame died on St Valentine's Day.

Michael Harrison suggests that, as this old lady had been a young woman when the Thompson-Bywaters murder case was on everyone's lips, she might have come to associate herself with her infamous namesake, and as time passed the irony of her own celibate life overwhelmed her. Perhaps her whole being yearned for something exciting to happen...perhaps she even wished she had been

that other Edith, who had known passion and notoriety, even though she paid the price with her life. The link with the murderess of the past, might have laid the foundations for a sudden tendency to go up in flames.

Or it may just be that the Joker likes a good laugh. One must remember that he is not very sophisticated; the broader the humour, the more obvious the pun, the greater his delight. (Perhaps his favourite pantomime is *Cinderella*.) To him, there is no such thing as a 'mere coincidence', although the connections may not be terribly obvious to we the victims, and possibly we might not find the jokes in the best of taste.

Not all cases of spontaneous combustion have dire results, however. The *Daily Express* of 3 February 1986 (and later the *Fortean Times*) carried the tale of chronic invalid Eddie Matthijs of Haalert in Belgium. One night his plaster madonna spontaneously combusted and Eddie's pain left him. His family noticed that: 'the scorchmarks on the wall behind the madonna resembled an image of Christ crowned with thorns, a dove and two devils. The left foot of the statue had escaped the flames. "She used this to crush the devils and cure my husband," said Mrs Matthijs. The shrine has had thousands of visitors, many of whom claim to see the faint images on the wall.'

There are two links with other cases of SHC here: a plastic statuette melted in the heat that finally destroyed suicide Billy Peterson, and the unburnt left foot seems to be almost a parody of the classic unburnt extremity in human combustion. What the connections *mean* is a matter for conjecture, but like us the gods have their private jokes. As the occultists say: 'As above, so below', and vice versa?

The High Command of the Great Conspiracy continue to deny the existence of SHC. It is a 'vulgar error' to believe in it. It is heresy. For how can our intelligent, sophisticated human species ever admit it doesn't even understand the true nature of *fire*?

4

▫ A DEADLY MASQUERADE ▫

THERE ARE MANY strange objects patrolling our sacred skies, piloted by a motley crew of silky-haired svelte Venusians (with a propensity for having sex with Earthlings), tiny humanoids with bulging foetus-like heads, the traditional Little Green Men with fair-skinned, red-haired lovelies. Their craft are usually, but not exclusively, flying saucers; but whatever their shape they must be shoddily made because people are always coming across grounded UFOs being mended by their weird occupants in forest glades or deserts.

Sometimes these 'contactees' are given rides in the repaired craft to obscure planets whose names are unfamiliar to astronomers. Until recent space probes revealed that Venus and Mars are uninhabitable, those two planets were often cited as the homeland of the UFOnauts. Frequently they give an object, as proof of their meeting, to the contactee, which on examination turns out to be only too terrestrial and mundane. And this object is often then taken back by the aliens before it can be inspected by anyone other than the contactee. Sometimes the aliens give the Earthling information about himself that proves his life has been closely monitored by them, and about the immediate future in local and world affairs – which comes true. The 'contactees' often suffer blinding headaches, black-outs and skin disorders as a direct result of their first meeting with the UFOnauts. They might start a cult based on their encounter, which is sometimes elevated to the status of a religion. But just when the cultists had obeyed their extraterrestrial lords' instructions to the letter – giving away their homes and belongings to take up residence in trees waiting for the arrival of the spaceships that will take them to a new, unpolluted planet...

Some 'jokes' are not very funny. These random sorties into human life by unreliable and heartless mavericks from non-existent planets are not new; only the trappings change, the better to deceive. Throughout history mankind has been plagued by the intrusions of gods, demons, angels, fairies – and now alleged aliens. Are they actually the same phenomenon, just keeping one step ahead of our current expectations?

The temptation to start a religion is great, especially when instructed to do so by God, or an angel, or both. But it must be resisted at all costs, or you will come to a grisly end. Your followers may not find themselves in an arena shared by ravenous lions, but financial ruin, mental instability, physical illness and a reputation in tatters makes the early Christians' fate seem like an easy way out. And the same vision that promised you marvels and wonders (then lets you down when it really matters), is the one that promised you a reward in heaven. One should pause for thought.

The existence of God is outside the scope of this book. We are more concerned with the *appearance* of heavenly beings to the Chosen, with intent to defraud. Consider the following:

THE ANSWER TO A PRAYER?

Two bearded men appeared in a glorious vision to farm-boy Joseph Smith in 1820, in Palmyra, New York. The area was in the middle of a religious revival, each sect proselytizing with incandescent fervour, but Smith was still undecided which of them to join. He had been praying for guidance the night before his vision and when one of the men pointed to the other, saying 'This is my beloved Son, hear ye him...' Smith knew that his quest was at an end.

The Answer had come to him; he had been

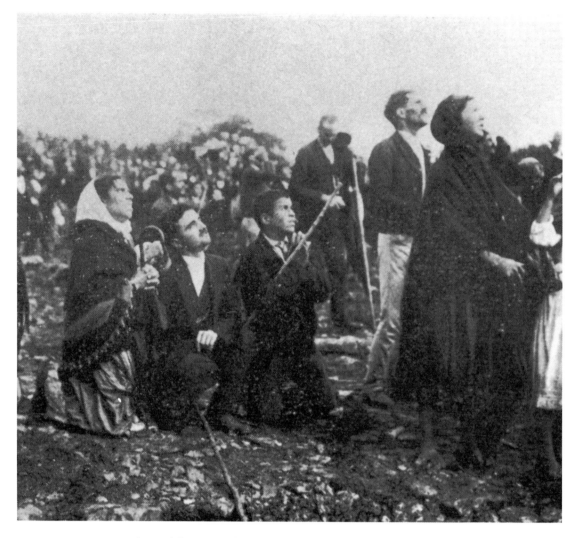

Members of the crowd that witnessed the strange behaviour of the sun
on 13 October 1917 at Fatima, Portugal. According to some reports it
'danced' in the heavens, fulfilling the prediction of the Virgin Mary to
some local child-visionaries. There is no doubt that these people, at least,
believed themselves to be witnessing a miracle. Most visions fulfil some
of their promises – at first.

chosen to reinstate the one and only Christian Church, which had, said the bearded man, died with the last Apostle. Joseph Smith, a humble lad, was to be the founder of the Church of Jesus Christ of Latter Day Saints, otherwise known as the Mormons. He was inspired to find some inscribed gold and bronze tablets hidden in a nearby hill, which being translated became *The Book of Mormon*, or the story of Jesus' visit to the people of the New World ('other sheep must I bring, which are not of this fold...') after his resurrection. The mysterious tablets were taken back by an angel when the translation was finished.

Smith became the Prophet of the new church, and quickly gathered around him a latter-day set of twelve apostles, and thousands of believers, some of whom emigrated from far-off Europe to join the Mormons.

Not unnaturally, the Latter Day Saints' monopoly of Christian truth was hotly disputed. Smith and his brother were murdered by a bizarre mob with painted faces. The movement then passed into the extraordinarily gifted hands of Brigham Young, 'the New Moses', who is mainly remembered for his enthusiastic espousal of the Mormon rule of polygamy, earning himself the nickname 'bring-'em-young - and - bring-'em-beautiful', (although few of his wives were either). Young took his faithful in covered wagons across the largely uncharted Wild West, guided, he believed, by God. The Mormons didn't know what they were looking for, but when they found it, he would tell them.

Schisms had wrought havoc with the wagon train; provisions were running low, as was morale. Young himself had been ill with a mysterious fever. The pathetic caravan of the new chosen halted before a dismal, hopeless waste of salt-flats. Had God let them down? Were they going to die of hunger or be murdered by Indians after all they had been through?

Suddenly restored to health, Young emerged from his wagon, overlooked the plain and said: 'This is the place.' For many, this was the last straw and their wagons rolled off into the sunset. The faithful were urged to buckle down and build, for 'the desert shall blossom as a rose'.

Before Salt Lake City rose to confound those of little faith, there was one more miracle. The Saints had toiled incredibly hard, building their makeshift City of God, draining the land and planting crops that were their only source of food and, more symbolically, a central act of faith. But yet another trial was visited upon them in the form of an anomalous swarm of locusts – a plague of Biblical dimensions – that fastened on their precious crops. Almost mad with despair they appealed to their prophet, Brigham Young. He prayed to

his God for mercy and there came, promptly and incredibly, an enormous flock of seagulls, that obligingly ate up the locusts before flying away. Salt Lake City is 1207 km (750 miles) from the coast.

But where the 'true Church' was concerned history was repeating itself, and time was running out for Mormon miracles. Today, the Church of Jesus Christ of Latter Day Saints has a thriving and successful missionary programme, but the religion has turned into a big corporation. 'Prophet' succeeds 'prophet' but inevitably they are wealthy businessmen, whose talks with God are not publicized and whose ability to heal the sick or to prophesy is nil. Mormonism is the American Dream personified, but it is no longer capable of marvels.

Joseph Smith has been revered as God's Chosen, and persecuted as an evil self-seeking fraud; perhaps he was neither, perhaps he was a victim. The Joker is fond of dressing up; he is master of a thousand disguises, all of them perfect for his chosen role. Joseph Smith had not joined the rush to the Methodists or the Quakers or the Lutherans; he hung back, imploring the powers that be for guidance – and that was his undoing. He had invited The Joker into his life. How could he have known that he was being set up just to be knocked down? He had prayed to God and God came in person to answer him.

Perhaps the ultimate sick joke is the indoctrination of all such religious contactees with the belief that they will reap the reward for their inevitable suffering on this earth in the heaven set aside for the Chosen. As Charles Fort would say: 'We have no data on this point', but it looks distinctly dubious.

THE THING IN THE TREES

Before she was locked up in a convent, Bernadette Soubirous was taken to see the building of the grotto that marked the site of her vision outside the little French town of Lourdes. Bernadette was very polite, but

The Blessed Virgin Mary in person. In Zeitoun, Egypt in 1968 some
Muslim workmen thought they saw a nun about to throw herself off the
roof of the nearby Coptic Orthodox Church, but when they fetched a
ladder the 'nun' bobbed out of reach.

remarked that the statue of The Lady looked
nothing like the entity she had seen. Not long
afterwards she developed a cancerous knee
and died in great pain.

In February 1858, fourteen-year-old

Bernadette Soubirous had discovered a strange
creature, apparently suspended among the
branches of a tree. It glowed, smiled and beck-
oned. The future Catholic saint did not, as in
the Hollywood version, fall enraptured to her

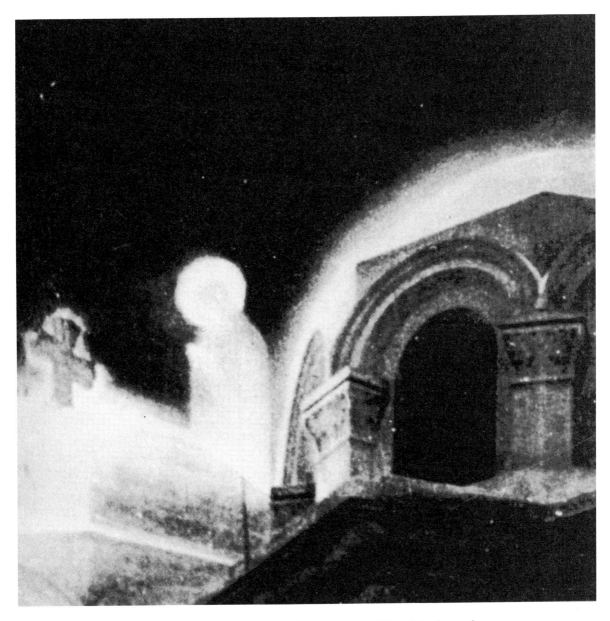

The vision obligingly remained on the roof – although it changed position – for ten days before it dissolved away. Was it a thoughtform created by the minds of believers, or some kind of hologram produced by person or creatures unknown? The vision gave no clue.

knees, but ran home to grab a bottle of holy water to throw at 'that thing', as she called the vision. She believed it to be a demon, sent by the Devil to lure her to her doom, and perhaps she was right.

The splash of holy water, however, did not make the vision disappear. Instead, it persisted and succeeded in befriending the young peasant girl, winning her confidence and bestowing extraordinary gifts on her – for a short time.

At first Bernadette was troubled, rather than ecstatic, about the visions and feared her lack of education might lead her to the wrong interpretation of the events. She took her extraordinary secret to the parish priest, the only man of letters she knew. History might have taken a different turn had he not been a fierce defendant of Mariolatry at a time when the status of the Virgin was being challenged within the Catholic Church. To him the identity of Bernadette's lady was obvious, and propagation of the vision would do his cause no harm, now she was proving herself by making miracles happen.

Every time the girl went to the appointed tree to keep her tryst with 'that thing' an increasingly large and hope-hungry crowd accompanied her, although no one but Bernadette saw anything unusual. Doubt now flung aside, the girl knelt before 'that thing' transfigured with ecstasy. Her eyes fixed on a point in the tree, she gave all the signs of listening intently; sometimes she murmured an answer, and occasionally actually put a question to the vision – for she had been primed by the Church authorities. To the vital question about her identity the vision answered 'I am the Immaculate Conception', a phrase Bernadette did not recognize, but which meant everything to the Mariologists.

When the rapture overwhelmed her, Bernadette fell into a trance in which she proved to be incombustible, holding her hand in the flame of a candle for fifteen minutes without injury. Then came the day when The Lady told her to eat the soil close to where she stood; despite a certain amount of derision Bernadette did as bidden. Later a stream welled up through the ground at that point, which proved to have miraculous curative powers. The grotto – complete with the dubious stone likeness of the Mother of God – was built at the site, and Bernadette went the way of those chosen by the strange beings that people our earth and raid our consciousness in order to guide our lives; she was taken to a convent and died not long afterwards.

Even in death the girl was marked out from her fellow beings; although not embalmed, her body did not decompose. Rather than stinking of putrefaction it gave off a sweet smell, 'the odour of sanctity'. When her body was disinterred twenty years after her death it looked as if the girl were merely sleeping, and the tumour had disappeared from her knee, resulting in a slight shortening of the afflicted leg.

Incorruptibility is an extraordinary phenomenon, and although most of the reports concern Catholic saints and martyrs, quite ordinary people have been found to have survived the ravages of the grave under circumstances that, if anything, should have hastened them. The corpses, as far as we know, are not reanimated, as in zombieism, but are miraculously preserved, often hundreds of years after their death. Sometimes they give off a clear, fragrant oil that is found to have curative properties, and the haunting 'odour of sanctity' that surrounded Bernadette's body.

THE SLEEP OF THE JUST

One is led, in the face of overwhelming evidence for incorruptibility, to add death to the list of human experiences that we just don't understand, but like to think we do. But even accepting that dead bodies lie there prettily exuding a dainty scent, we ask what is the point? In many cases the miracle serves to reinforce the legends surrounding that person's life and works, and keep his or her name associated with marvels and miracle cures centuries after their death. The odd nonentity who has been found to lie perfectly preserved and pliable inside a rotten coffin in swampy land, may have had an intensely holy inner life that was thus rewarded in the privacy of the grave. But somehow, such apparently random phenomena suggest a mistake. Like 11-month-old Peter Seaton (page 70) who seemed to have got in the way of the 'Fire from Heaven' and met his end in a ball of flame perhaps not intended for him, these corpses may well be preserved by the fickleness of fate – perhaps as

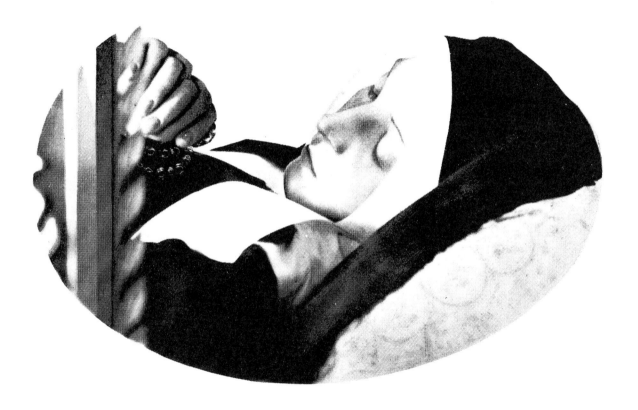

Bernadette of Lourdes lies dead, miraculously uncorrupted by the grave,
surrounded by a strange, sweet scent – 'the odour of sanctity'.
Incorruptibility is not, however, the monopoly of the saints. In any case,
the phenomenon is particularly provocative: is death something else we
just don't understand?

an experiment for a Learner God? Unlike SHC the 'gift' of incorruptibility apparently does no harm to the recipient, but one could argue that it does precious little good, besides top up the level of hysteria in the believers.

We are being played with, but if it's any comfort we could be educational toys...

At the other extreme comes the case of John Bennett, a fifty-one-year-old Liverpudlian whose 'horrifically decomposed' body was found in his flat, where he lived alone, by the caretaker in 1985. The body was so far advanced in decay that pathologist James Burns told the inquest that 'I cannot even ascertain the cause of death.' Yet Bennett had been seen three days before his body had been found, and had apparently attended a family christening only the week before. Had he died of unknown causes weeks before, as the state of his body indicated, and a solid-seeming ghost gone about its business in the locality? Or was it, as the *Fortean Times* suggests, 'an interesting counterpoint to those tales of miraculous incorruption...'

At this point it is tempting to slink back into the folds of the Great Conspiracy, with tail between our legs. But we know too much to be allowed back in. We know fewer answers than are claimed by the Conspirators but we are beginning to frame the right questions and have learned to be on our guard against the depredations of the Joker, although it seems as if swift retribution may follow our insurrection. Freedom is never easy; to recognize that Man knows so little about fire, or life or death, comes hard to our sophisticated species. But escaping from the smug preconceptions of the Great Conspiracy is truly educative; we know what we don't know, which is just about everything.

If a consensus of opinion is the only mechanism that keeps things in their place (it generally stops levitation from happening and maintains, for example, a table in the shape to which we have become accustomed) then the universe really is, as Eddington said, 'made of mind-stuff.' But whose mind is it that has created the world, and all things in it?

THE GOOD DIE YOUNG

The Cosmic Joker is a master of disguise, appearing to us clothed in the trappings of our own predilections, the better to further his plan, or practical joke...Joseph Smith saw a Victorian-looking God and Jesus after a bout of intense prayer. The young and the malleable are easy prey for the powers-that-be, as stories of poltergeist possession and visions of the Virgin show. Bernadette showed spirit by believing her lady to be a demon, but under pressure from believers, she crumbled. The miracle cures surrounding the grotto remain controversial, but significantly, they are few and far between. Like Mormonism, a visit to Lourdes is comforting, but hopes are too often raised just to be dashed. Joseph Smith and Bernadette Soubirous, like many other visionaries, died young. (What would have happened if they had refused to acknowledge their visions is, of course, hypothetical. Perhaps they would have lived out their natural span, happy in their obscurity, or perhaps there would have been two more cases of SHC thousands of miles apart?)

Interestingly, Smith's home in Palmyra, New York, was just a few miles from Hydesville, which was to become the birthplace of Spiritualism. Perhaps paranormal phenomena are 'place-centred', just waiting to be triggered by the approach of the right person?

Bernadette's vision appeared in a tree, Smith's bearded men came to him in a wood. Man has always known that shrubbery attracts creatures from other planes of existence who, according to the fashionable belief of the time, sometimes can be seen as fairies, sprites, nymphs or gnomes (or 'that thing', God, and Jesus?). Since earliest times woods and forests were to be avoided, especially at night, and not merely for fear of falling prey to medieval muggers. The shadows that loom in the woods are waiting to confront you or make you mad with panic...(The word 'panic' comes from 'Pan', mischievous god of the great outdoors.) The countryside is crowded with a paranormal host.

THE CASE OF THE COTTINGLEY FAIRIES

Two young girls who successfully championed the cause of fairies for many years, against all the odds, were Elsie Wright and her cousin Frances Griffiths. As children they had allegedly taken some photographs of fairies capering about the trees and bushes near the Wrights' home at Cottingley, West Yorkshire, in the last days of the First World War. By now, their confession to having faked the pictures is well-known, although of course it had been suspected since Sir Arthur Conan Doyle had first publicized them. Fairies do not exist, so how can they be photographed?

What is less well-known is the girls' reason for their hoax: they often saw fairies and were annoyed that they couldn't capture them on film, so they faked them. Moreover, Frances went to her grave maintaining that *one* of the famous photographs was real...

On 9 November 1918, eleven-year-old Frances sent a letter to a friend back in South Africa, where she had lived most of her young life. Among the schoolgirlish scrawl was an astounding statement:

> I am learning French, Geometry, Cookery and Algebra at school now. Dad came home from France the other week after being there for ten months, and we all think the war will be over in a few days. We are going to get our flags to hang upstairs in our bedroom. I am sending two photos, both of me, one of me in a bathing costume in our back yard, Uncle Arthur took that, while the other one is me with some fairies up at the beck, Elsie took that one...How are Teddy and Dolly?

The enclosed photograph was of young Frances Griffiths staring determinedly at the camera behind a troupe of cavorting fairies, all winged and all female. Frances had scribbled on the back: 'Elsie and I are very friendly with the beck fairies. It is funny I never used to see them in Africa. It must be too hot for them there.'

The two cousins claimed to have seen fairies around the 'beck' (the local term for stream) as an everyday occurrence. Certainly at the time of this letter there was no intention of seeking fame or notoriety with the enclosed photograph. They seemed to think of it in the light of a snap for the family album, like the picture of the little girl in her bathing costume in the back yard.

Elsie had borrowed her father's camera on a hot Saturday afternoon in July 1917, to take a picture of Frances and the beck fairies, and Mr Wright developed the plate later that day. The anomalous white shapes that gradually emerged in the foreground were first taken to be sandwich papers littering up the grass, or some kind of bird. Elsie piped up that they were fairies, but Mr Wright took no notice. When it was Frances' turn with the Midg quarter-plate a month later, she managed to capture Elsie with a gnome. Arthur Wright questioned the two closely but they stuck to their story; they had just taken pictures of what had been there. Nevertheless, borrowing the camera was banned from then on.

Being an ordinary, agreeable Conspirator, Arthur Wright behaved predictably when faced with the impossible. He and his wife Polly combed the area around the beck and searched the girls' rooms for tell-tale signs of fraud, but they came away empty handed. The pictures certainly had novelty-value; some prints were made to show to neighbours.

Polly, however, was a believer – something often played down in the Cottingley story, and Fate (whatever or whoever that is) was greedy for her contribution. She was a member of the Theosophical Society, which had been founded in the late-nineteenth century by the highly controversial and flamboyant Madame Helena Blavatsky, allegedly under the guidance of the mysterious 'masters' from the

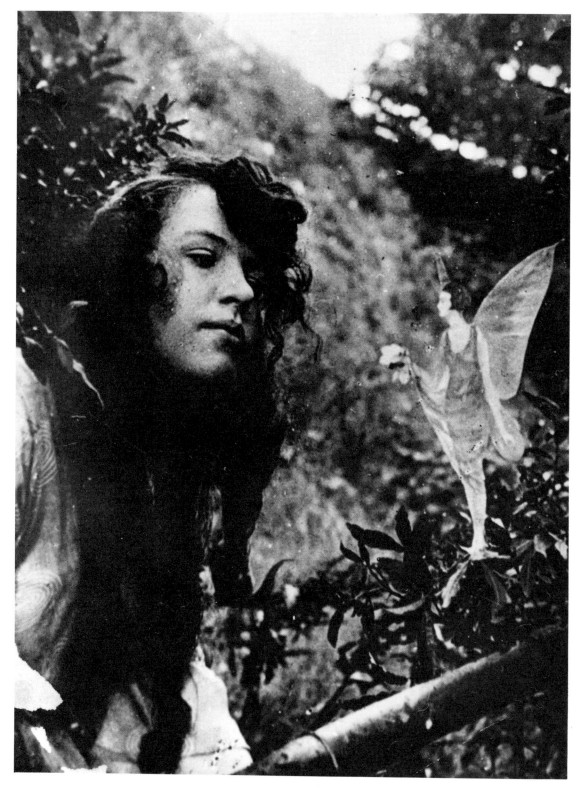

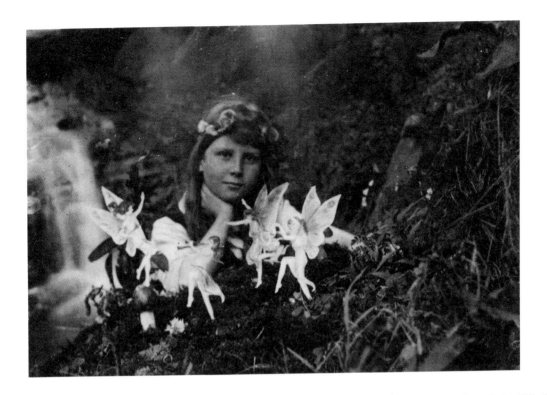

Left Elsie Wright soberly views a fairy close to the 'beck' (stream) in Cottingley, Yorkshire in 1921. The photograph was taken by her cousin Frances Griffiths, whose own fairy photograph (*above*) began the Cottingley Fairy controversy that continues today. For over sixty years the two women maintained a poker-faced attitude to their fairies, despite ridicule from all quarters. Elsie's mother Polly, a staunch Theosophist and believer in fairies, first made the photographs known and within a few months Sir Arthur Conan Doyle, latterly a champion of Spiritualism, became involved. Many took this to be a sure sign of the great man's senility. Two batches of fairy photographs were taken, including one of a dancing gnome (*right*); all of which looked suspiciously like cardboard cut-outs – but even computer enhancement failed to reveal tell-tale string. It was only in the 1980s that the two old ladies chucklingly admitted to their hoax – but it was a confession with a difference; they had faked the pictures, they said, because of their frustration at being unable to capture on film *what they often saw* around the beck at Cottingley. They chose to reveal the true story to their friend Joe Cooper, retired sociology lecturer, because he believes in fairies and Frances went to her grave maintaining that one of the photographs was genuine. Sceptics will choose to remember only the confession; inevitably, however, the truth is much more complex.

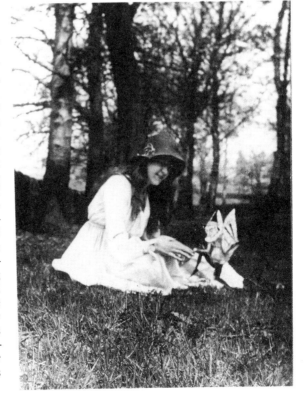

East. The Society flourished in an atmosphere of belief and excitement in the impossible. It was at a local Theosophical Society meeting – a lecture on fairy life – that Polly confided to others that her daughter and niece had taken photographs of fairies. Within months the news had spread to Edward L. Gardner, a leading Theosophist and expert on fairy lore.

Fate was on good form; at the same time as Gardner was enthusing over sharpened prints of the Cottingley beck fairies, Sir Arthur Conan Doyle was researching an article on fairies, which was to be published in the *Strand Magazine* at the end of the year. Gardner's 'find' naturally came to his ears.

'SHE DID NOT TAKE ONE FLYING...'

Conan Doyle will always be best remembered as the creator of the cynical, coldly-reasoning Sherlock Holmes, but in his later years the genius of the Edinburgh doctor had become focused on the cause of Spiritualism. It had lost him many friends; the word even went about that Conan Doyle was senile. The case of the Cottingley fairies clinched matters for the sceptics.

His was still a name to be reckoned with, however, and his involvement in this case attracted a great deal of publicity. But even Doyle was wary of the photographs at first. He sought other opinions; leading light of the Society for Psychical Research Sir Oliver Lodge, pronounced them fakes, although a clairvoyant's only strong impressions were more concerned with the character of Gardner's photoprinter, Mr Snelling, than with the background to the pictures themselves. (Snelling himself was described with striking accuracy.)

But obviously the girls were central to the issue – perhaps they were gifted mediums? Doyle sent Gardner up north to meet them and investigate the magic beck.

Gardner found the area distinctly promising and the girls and the Wrights seemingly honest, but he did not manage to capture a

single fairy or gnome with his own camera. Doyle had gone off to Australia to give a lecture tour on Spiritualism, leaving Gardner to cope as best he could with the media storm that followed the breaking of the story.

On 5 January 1921 *Truth* stated: 'For the true explanation of these fairy photographs what is wanted is not a knowledge of occult phenomena but a knowledge of children.' The *City News* later in the month said: 'It seems at this point that we must either believe in the almost incredible mystery of the fairy or in the almost incredible wonders of faked photographs.'

They were all, however, out of date. For in the school holidays in the summer of 1920 the girls had taken three more fairy photographs: one showing a distinctly two-dimensional fairy with fashionably bobbed hair, offering a flower to thirteen-year-old Elsie, and one showing a 'fairy bower', in a sort of cobwebby – or perhaps ectoplasmic – cocoon suspended from the branches of a tree (which was greatly exclaimed over by Conan Doyle). The third photograph of the batch shows Frances apparently moving back from a leaping fairy – only captured jumping on camera at its fifth leap, according to the girls.

Gardner, masking his excitement as usual with fussy attention to detail, took himself and two loaded cameras once again up to Cottingley in August 1920. He explained simply how they worked and then accompanied Elsie and Frances as they went about the beck, attempting to 'tice the fairies' to be photographed. Gardner wrote later: 'I knew it was essential they should feel free and unhampered and have no burden of responsibility. If nothing came of it all, I told them they were not to mind a bit.'

But again, for friends of the impossible, by far the most telling comments of the time came from Polly Wright, Elsie's mother, who wrote of their first day of the session: 'I went to my sister's for tea and left them to it. When I got back they had only managed two fairies, I was disappointed.' Two days later she added this astonishing postscript to a note about the girls' photographic experiments: 'P.S. She did not

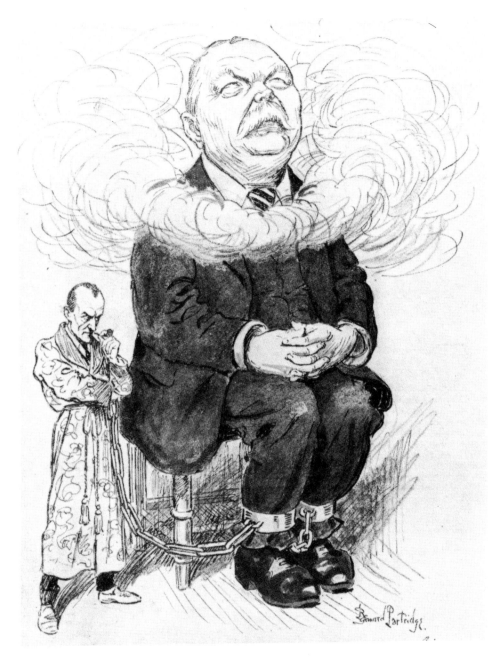

A contemporary view of the aging Sir Arthur Conan Doyle: while his head is swathed in the mists of Spiritualism, he remains manacled to his coldly logical creation, Sherlock Holmes. Arthur Wright, father of one of the Cottingley girls, never got over his disillusionment with Conan Doyle's belief in the fairies, being cheated 'by our Elsie – and her at the bottom of the class!' The news of the Yorkshire fairies came just at the right time for the great writer, however, coinciding with the research for his book *The Coming of The Fairies*.

take one flying after all.' Perhaps it was Polly's total belief that kept the mischief alive — paranormal or not?

Those three plates showing fairies among the Cottingley foliage were nevertheless created somehow, and were packed with loving care by Arthur Wright to be dispatched to London. Many years later Elsie was to repeat during an interview for Yorkshire Television that: 'Father had nothing to do with it...he knew nothing about it.' But at that stage she was studiedly evasive about her own part in the case.

Arthur had been privately disturbed by the affair. For one thing, a cherished dream had been shattered; the creator of the great Sherlock Holmes had been cheated 'by our Elsie, and her at the bottom of the class!'

ELEMENTALS, MY DEAR

Doyle seized upon the second batch of fairy photographs to illustrate another *Strand Magazine* article in 1921, and used them as the foundation for his book *The Coming of the Fairies* (1922).

For someone of his learning and understanding, Doyle behaved as if possessed, for anyone with the slightest familiarity with fairies knows that they tend to deceive, like all the Joker's creatures. Traditionally, in rural areas, 'will-o-the-wisps' bobbed about deadly bogs enticing the unwary to their doom; and the true nature of 'fairy gold' is legendary. Although he acknowledged their elemental nature — and by implication their ability to change their shape to accommodate the beliefs of the beholder — Doyle was too steeped in Spiritualism to see the underlying sameness of apparently different phenomena. As always, this led to his undoing.

In that same August, Geoffrey Hodgson, a medium with a particular interest in nature spirits, took the journey up to Cottingley. Many years later both the girls, by then old ladies, admitted somewhat gleefully that they had 'played Mr Hodgson along.' They claimed

to see fairies, but so did he. In fact, the 'dancing fairies of Cottingley' (*sic*) figure in his *Fairies at Work and Play* (1922):

A bright radiance shines out over the field, visible to us sixty yards away. It is due to the arrrival of a group of fairies. They are under the control of a superior fairy who is very autocratic and definite in her orders, holding unquestioned command. They spread themselves out into a gradually widening circle around her and, as they do so, a soft glow shines over the grass. Since two minutes ago, when they swung high over the tree tops and down into the field, the circle has spread to approximately twelve feet in width and is wonderfully radiant with light. Each member of this fairy band is connected to the directing fairy, who is in the centre and slightly above them, by a stream of light. These streams are of different shades of yellow deepening to orange, they meet in the centre merging in her aura, and there is a constant flow backwards and forwards along them. The form produced by this is something like an inverted fruit dish with the central fairy as the stem, and the lines of light, which flow in the graceful even curve, forming the sides of the bowl.

Their continued activities were producing an ever-increasing complexity of form, when time, unhappily, forced us to depart.

Years afterwards, Elsie was to look at a photograph of the two girls with Hodgson, and exclaim: 'Look at that — fed up with fairies!'

Over the years, the fairy photographs have been subjected to increasingly sophisticated scrutiny, including computer enhancement which seemed, perhaps — just possibly — to prove to James 'the Amazing' Randi and other cohorts of the Great Conspiracy, that the figures were suspended from nearly invisible strings. (Just where two little girls from the outskirts of Bradford would have found invisible string in 1917 is not explained.) He also remarked that the fairy figures in the original photograph bore a striking resemblance to the illustrations in the 1914 *Princess Mary's Gift Book*, which was very popular among young girls...

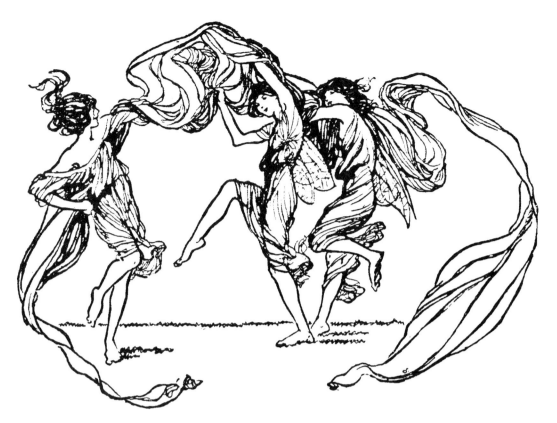

A plate from *Princess Mary's Gift Book*, a popular possession of young girls in 1914. The suspicions of years were confirmed in the 1980s when it was revealed that the Cottingley fairies were cardboard cut-outs based on these illustrations and propped up with hatpins.

FALLING INTO THE TENDER TRAP

After nearly seventy years of conjecture, the mystery of the Cottingley fairies was finally solved, or so it seemed. The weekly publication *The Unexplained* had carried three articles on the case, written by retired sociology lecturer Joe Cooper, who had befriended Elsie and Frances over the years. But after the staff received an audio tape of a chat between the old ladies and Joe, a fourth piece was quickly scheduled, that was to be entitled 'Cottingley: at last the truth.'

The photographs were hoaxes. The fairies were, as many had suspected, merely cut-outs based on the illustrations in *Princess Mary's Gift Book* and propped up among the grass by hat pins – except for one. Frances was to maintain to her dying day that the fifth and final picture of the 'fairy bower' was genuine: 'I saw these fairies building up in the grasses and just

aimed the camera and took a photograph.' She often mentioned a mental block that obscured her memory of the fairy photographs; Elsie had no such problem, she bluntly declared they were all fakes. But they were, they both asserted, created in order to show an unbelieving adult world what they *often* saw around the beck at Cottingley. As Frances said: 'I became so used to them that unless they did something unusual I just ignored them'.

The old ladies had weathered many a critical storm over the years and had become experts in evading the truth of the affair. Conan Doyle, Hodgson, Gardner and their own family were all gone so they spoke out. Joe Cooper succeeded where many others had failed because he believes in fairies. Elsie and Frances knew they had a friend in Joe and accorded him the ultimate accolade of telling him the truth. If he trapped them into revealing all it was the tenderest of traps, and an opportunity to confess that perhaps they had been waiting for. They had managed to keep up the hoax all those years by reiterating the original story with deadpan expressions, and letting their audience make of it what they will. Elsie frequently said: 'I would rather we were thought of as solemn-faced comediennes.'

FAIRIES FOR ALL

Since eliciting the Cottingley scoop in 1983 Joe Cooper has unremittingly pursued fairies through the fieldwork of his three flourishing evening classes in Psychic Studies in the Leeds area. Recently he sent me a summary of his findings:

> Belief in fairies hinges upon an individual's reading and experience. Few people have seen or heard them and the literature on Tinkerbell is usually only associated with childhood; as we grow older we 'put aside childish things' as they say – and that includes a belief in fairies. To confess in adulthood to such a belief automatically labels one as an oddball. I have to confess to being such a creature.
>
> I am fairly certain that more people have seen, and indeed played and conversed with, fairies in their childhood than is commonly supposed. I have perhaps a dozen quite lengthy tapes from very well-balanced older ladies who recall such happenings. And over the last few weeks (November-December 1986) I have recorded two further accounts: one from a modish seventeen-year-old who saw a fairy on her bedside cabinet, and another from a seven-year-old who really did see a fairy at the bottom of the garden, standing on the stone wall.
>
> I myself have never seen or heard the sprites but once, after one of my lectures on the subject, pussy willow buds mysteriously arranged themselves on the polished floor beneath the lectern; nobody had approached the area during the five minutes between the end of the talk and the discovery of the pattern. And, after our 'Tinkerbell '86' expedition to look for evidence of fairies, which was covered by the *Guardian* and the *York-*

shire Post, I was interviewed by Guy Michelmore and the sound unaccountably wavered from time to time. Later the same day I was having a preliminary discussion before being interviewed on Radio Two, and a crossed line interrupted our conversation – it was a deep voice talking of Pan and the fairies! And later in that week I was on a phone-in on local radio and the device holding calls went, unaccountably, haywire. All 'coincidence'? I doubt it.

> Some of my taped accounts, honestly given I would say, are bizarre to say the least; a sandwich-snatching gnome on a Gibraltar hillside; a fairy rescued from a spider's web in New Zealand; Devas sixty feet high by the side of trees, and a gnome appearing to a little boy in an attic, repeating his name over and over in a tinkling voice: 'Cyril...Cyril...Cyril...'

> On our summer expedition we heard two fairy bells and one of our members saw dark earth spirits scurrying along an old pathway. Another heard the sound of high fairy talk in a flower bed – in common with others, the capacity to see fairies in her childhood had given way to hearing them only in her adulthood. In another case the lady now 'saw bright geometrical shapes' after she grew out of seeing fairies in more detail as a girl.

> The subject thus awaits further scrutiny. It is on the grounds of evidence and prudent argument that the matter will be settled; meanwhile we believers await the evidence relating to Fraud, Fancy or Fiction from the sceptics with interest. To date, nothing substantial has been forthcoming to counter the results of our pioneering fieldwork.

> Yet for me Tink is light of heart and yawns at such boring discussion. She much prefers me to play a syncopated rhythm on my ukelele, as did Frances of Cottingley when we were trying to write a book together. But she's gone now, and all I have left of our collaboration is the tape of her experiences with the nature spirits.

> Perhaps the day is dawning when others may take her testimony seriously...

It is more likely that Frances will be remembered for her confession; her statement of belief in the fairies she saw conveniently ignored. Sceptics always prefer a neat case, one that is very firmly closed.

THE EYE OF THE BEHOLDER

Edward Gardner had developed a theory about the true nature of fairies that seems to accord with the huge variety of human experience of them. They have no particular shape intrinsically but can adopt almost any form, appearing:

> To be influenced from two directions – the physical outer conditions prevailing, and an inner intelligent urge...What determines the shape assumed, and how the transformation is effected, is not clear. One may speculate as to the influence of human thought, individual or in the mass, and quite probably the explanation when found will include this influence as a factor.

In other words fairies look the way they do because something in our minds helps to shape them. It goes beyond individual predilection, although this is a powerful force in shaping the curious bundle of energy and intelligence that presents itself to us. Our collective unconscious may select archetypal images and project them on to the raw elemental force, producing the materialization of our choice. It may not always be a comforting creation – demons and threatening aliens may sometimes result – but it is literally the thought that counts. Creatures and beings that we suppose only exist in our dreams or in folklore can rise up to confront us as we go about our daily business with a vividness and impact that, not surprisingly, can threaten our sanity. In this dramatic way they reach straight into the centre of our being.

Air Marshal Sir Victor Goddard added to Gardner's theory in a public lecture given at Caxton Hall in London on 3 May 1969:

> The astral world of illusion, which is greatly inhabited by illusion-prone spirits, is well known for its multifarious imaginative activities and exhortations. Seemingly some of its denizens are eager to exemplify principalities and powers. Others pronounce upon morality, spirituality, Deity etc. All of these astral exponents who invoke human consciousness may be sincere, but many of their theses may be framed to propagate some special phantasm...or simply to astonish and disturb the gullible for the devil of it.

In being 'illusion-prone' these spirits more than meet Man halfway, for he is himself an excellent source of fodder for propagating any and every gospel, cult or creed. Sometimes it pleases the elementals to lead us into temptation with golden promises and then sit back while we struggle all alone, wretched and despised, a martyr for a cause based on nothing – but which had seemed to promise everything. The meteoric rise and fall of Joan of Arc, one of history's most famous visionaries, is a cautionary tale to those who let angels into their lives.

APPOINTED BY GOD

Joan was thirteen years old when she first heard her voices. It was a hot summer's day and she was in the garden at Domrèmy, alone. A voice came out of the air from the direction of the church, 'with an accompanying brightness', and at first she was afraid. But gradually she came to live for her voices, which claimed to be those of the Archangel Michael, St Catherine of Alexandria and St Margaret of Antioch. They exhorted her to be a good girl, to remain a virgin and to prepare herself for a great destiny.

After she had led the victorious French army to raise the siege of Orleans on 8 May 1429 the voices began to address her as 'The Daughter of God'. So far everything they had prophesied for her had come true, against incredible odds. This little girl even had to learn to ride a horse before beginning her military career, but there must have been an aura of the Chosen about her, for thousands of men to march under her banner...

She so impressed the Dauphin that he bestowed on her a black charger and a white suit of armour, and appointed her the leader of his forces. Her voices had told her his secret prayer and when she repeated it to him verbatim, he was persuaded that she had been sent to him by God.

The psychic powers conferred on her by the saints enabled her to find lost or hidden objects of great symbolic value; her battle sword, she declared, was buried behind the altar at St Catherine's Church at Fierbois. It was found there, although no one had known of its existence. She helped to find a pair of lost gloves that had been gifts for the guests at the Dauphin's coronation at Rheims. She simply knew where they were; her voices told her.

In May 1430 while attempting to relieve the siege of Compiègne, she was knocked off her horse and taken to Beaurevoir, and then Rouen, prisons. Her trial began before the Vice-Inquisitor of France in March 1431. She was charged with blasphemy and heresy – and witchcraft.

Joan was faithful to her voices, despite the dank and disgusting conditions in which she was kept, chained at her waist as well as at her feet, with a constant watch by jailers who indulged themselves in round-the-clock sexual harassment of this strange girl in men's clothing. She fell ill and grew confused in her mind.

When she was shown her scaffold being built and urged to recant, she suddenly made a confession, agreeing that her heresies included: 'worshipping evil spirits and invoking them'. Her captors were jubilant; a wave of agonized disillusionment spread throughout the ranks of her defeated army. Her sentence was transmuted to life imprisonment, but when the judges visited her cell a few days afterwards, they found a very different Joan waiting to face them. Still in her male attire, she told them that 'since Thursday her voices had told her that she had done great wrong to God in confessing that what she had done was not well done.'

Who knows what she had been promised, what salvation in this world or the next when the sweet bright light came to visit her dungeon? She was condemned to be burnt alive and went to the stake obdurately in male dress on 30 May 1431. She was nineteen years old.

They tied her to the stake on a specially-constructed high platform in the market place at Rouen, and lit the huge pile of wooden faggots under it. An enormous crowd packed the square; many of them embittered soldiers from her defeated army, some perhaps still hoping for a miraculous escape for the Daughter of God. But the flames licked at her feet as at those of many a martyr before and since, and her only gesture was to kiss the cross she grasped and murmur 'Jesu...'

When the ashes were raked over her heart was found untouched by the fire.

BEDEVILLED BY RUMOUR

The Catholic Church finally recognized Joan's sanctity in 1920 when she was canonized. The decision to let her into the exclusive club of saints had not been easy, for her story had been bedevilled by rumours of demonic possession, even of pacts with the Devil himself.

Her enemies in battle had certainly believed her to be, as the Duke of Bedford wrote to the English king: 'a disciple...of the fiend...that used fals enchauntments and sorcerie, and which...nought only lessed...the nombre of your peuple there, but as well withdrowe the courage of the remnant, in marvellous wyse...'

She had refused to say the Lord's prayer at her trial, perhaps because in her weakened state she might have stammered, and that would have been taken as a sure sign that she was a witch, but there was still the possibility that she refused because she really was a witch...After all, was she not influenced by the notorious satanist Gilles de Rais, who was a Captain in her army at Orleans? (Her supporters point out that his mass torture and murder of children took place after her death, but surely St Michael could have detected the presence of great evil in the army marching under his banner?)

Beside the Enchanted Tree

At her trial Joan was also accused of consorting with 'evil spirits called fairies' who frolicked in the fountain near an ancient tree, 'the tree enchanted by fairies of Bourlement', near Domrèmy. In the Acts of Accusation it was said:

> Joan was wont to frequent the fountain and the tree, mostly at night, sometimes during the day; particularly, so as to be alone, at hours when in church the divine office was being celebrated. When dancing she would turn around the tree and the fountain, then would hang on the boughs garlands of different herbs and flowers, made by her own hand, dancing and singing while, before and after, certain songs and verses and invocations, spells and evil arts. And the next morning the chaplets of flowers would no longer be found there.

This calumny has frequently been dismissed as merely the charming girlish observance of a rural custom, but no matter what her intention was, the effect was to lay her wide open to the elemental energy that perpetually waits in ambush. Everything was right for a psychic attack:

She was pubescent and given to wandering rural areas alone. She left pretty garlands of flowers as tribute to the fairies who were said to live in the fountain by the enchanted tree – local belief reinforcing the power of the elemental presence. She was fervently patriotic at a time when France was suffering humiliations at the hands of the Prussians and the English. She was uneducated and very religious. And she was available.

The saints who came to call were familiar names to her, and St Michael is 'Lord Protector and Archangel of the Sun', commonly pictured as a soldier of God in shining armour, his hands folded on a sword of fire. The symbolism was perfect. The voices were preceded by a glowing light, as are most victims', be they of God, or of aliens in UFOs. And although Joan was to remain mainly clairaudient, the saints did show themselves to her on one occasion: 'I saw them with the eyes of my body, as plainly as I see you; and when they left me, I wept, and longed for them to take me away with them.' The image of their faces remained etched on her memory, and the apparitions had given off a sweet scent, 'the odour of sanctity'.

They told her amazing and unlikely things that proceeded to come true: certainly her meteoric rise as a military leader defies all normal explanation. Her voices urged her on, then she was knocked off her horse and taken prisoner like anyone else. The shock must have been intense, but all during her trial – which was punctuated with threats of hideous torture – she stood by her angelic voices, believing they would so honour her. Yet when she saw them building the scaffold, she faltered for the first time. Had her voices forsaken her? She confessed to anything put to her by her captors. It was then that the saints visited her cell to make her retract and put a seal on her fate. Perhaps it is worth noting it was not St Michael's name she uttered in her torment, but that of Jesus.

Her unburnt heart might be taken as a sign of incorruptibility, although that of poet and atheist Percy Bysshe Shelley also survived his funeral pyre. Even so, incorruptibility is only a posthumous honour, and as much a comfort to a living girl enduring the agonies of the stake as the knowledge that it was below freezing in Siberia.

After her canonization in 1920 she was declared the patron saint of France, but twenty years later the jackboots still echoed all over her land. One expects better from the saints.

The Master Manipulators

Visionaries are so persuaded of the righteousness of their cause that nothing will stand in their way. The master manipulators, the cun-

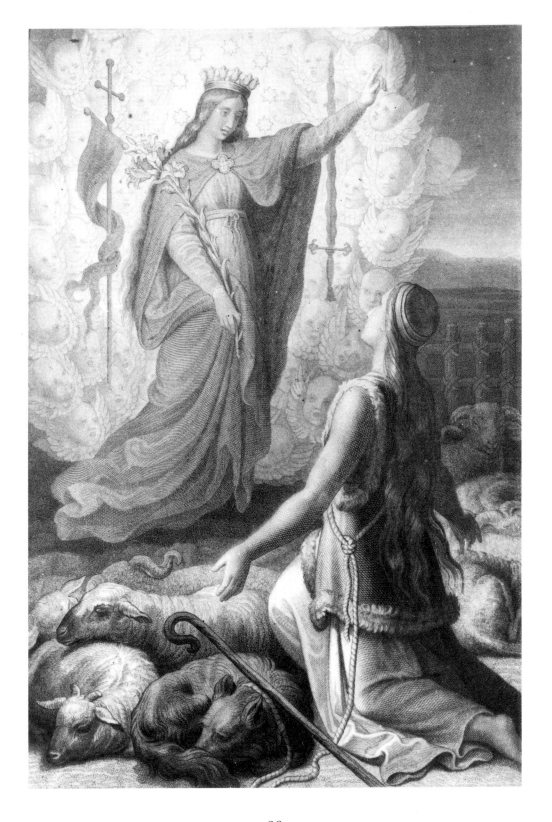

ning elementals, demand nothing less than total obedience.

Today's UFOnauts choose their messiahs from all walks of life, but it still helps not to be particularly well read. Anyone with a nodding acquaintance with the classics might think twice before taking orders from a creature that calls itself 'Xeno' (which is Greek for 'no-one') and, as John F. Keel points out in *Operation Trojan Horse*:

> Thousands of mediums, psychics, and UFO contactees have been receiving mountains of messages from 'Ashtar' in recent years. Mr Ashtar represents himself as a leader in the great intergalactic councils which hold regular meetings on Jupiter, Venus, Saturn and many planets known to us. But Ashtar is not a new arrival. Variations of this name, such as Astaroth, Ashar, Asharoth, etc., appear in demonological literature throughout history, both in the Orient and the Occident. Mr Ashtar has been around a very long time, posing as assorted gods and demons and now, in the modern phase, as another glorious spaceman.

A cult called the 'Light Affiliates', based in Burnaby, British Columbia and active in the 1960s, had the singular distinction of answering to a space being called Ox-Ho, and one of their number had the honour of being renamed 'Truman Merit'. (Here again names are seen as of enormous significance. Just as newcomers to monastic orders adopt a religious name, and Annie Owen Morgan became 'Katie King' for her earthly mission, so UFO contactees affect a change of name to indicate that a new phase of their lives has begun.) The Light Affiliates were given a

A highly romanticized representation of Joan of Arc beholding the vision of St Margaret of Antioch. The young French girl was, in fact, mainly *clairaudient* – she heard, rather than saw – paranormal entities, who claimed to be three of her favourite saints. Her short and spectacular life followed a pattern familiar with visionaries: their initial experience is closely followed by miracles then their powers desert them, and they are left alone to die horribly as martyrs.

number of minor prophecies that came true, and were told that the day of judgement would take place on 22 November 1969...

Ludicrous though they may seem to most people, some of the UFO cults have the potential to be downright dangerous. Leading UFOlogist Dr Jacques Vallée has developed the 'control system theory', which he first propounded in *The Invisible College*: 'UFOs are the means through which man's concepts are being arranged...I suggest that it is human belief that is being controlled', while psychical researcher and author D. Scott Rogo stated:

> UFO abductions are physically real events. But they are dramas materialised into three-dimensional space for us by the Phenomenon [the controlling intelligence]. They are dreams that the Phenomenon made come to life in very frightening vividness...Once someone has entered into psychic contact with the Phenomenon the link may become permanent, and reactivate periodically.

URI'S UFO LINK

At the start of his international career as a metal-bending psychic, Uri Geller met Dr Andrija Puharich, an Hungarian-born American inventor whose presence seems to act as a catalyst for the psychic abilities of others. In particular, Puharich used hypnosis as a channel to put the subject in touch with 'the Nine', space-beings on an intergalactic peace mission. During one hypnosis session in 1971 Geller told how he had awakened, aged three, to find a disc-shaped object hovering over him, which knocked him down to the ground with a beam of light. At this point Geller's recollections were interrupted by the metallic monotone of a space-being who announced that the earth was about to embark on the ultimate war and that Geller had been programmed all those years before to avert the coming disaster.

On coming out of his trance Geller himself remembered nothing of this, and the recording of the session disappeared. Later Puharich witnessed the young Israeli climb on board a

UFO, which he photographed enthusiastically. The film vanished from his camera.

Today Uri Geller explains the sensational reports of his relationships with UFOs as part of an elaborate childhood fantasy – he often looked at the sky and *wished*...

Since his involvement with Geller, Dr Puharich has worked with other potential psychics, such as Greta Keller and medium Phyllis Schlemmer, both of whom acted as channels for alien beings and who began to exhibit extraordinary abilities, such as precognition, metal-bending and bodily transfiguration. Another of Puharich's 'Chosen', Bobby Horne, stormed out of his guru's laboratory when it dawned on him that the 'space-beings' seemed (in Colin Wilson's phrase): 'to be led by the spirit of W.C. Fields!'

Just who is being duped and by whom? And is there a sinister purpose behind the space beings' gifts of psychic abilities?

Geller had a lucky escape, and continues to survive the slings and arrows that tend to dog the fortunes of those who outrage rationalism, but the fact remains that, if he was not born psychic, he certainly is now. Puharich's part in his life may never be precisely analysed.

CONTROLLING THE CONTROLS

So are we totally at the mercy of the fairies, demons, angels, saints and aliens who lie in wait for us like muggers of the mind? Do these intelligences have a purpose for humanity and if so, are we being used for good or evil? That very much depends on us. For even if, as the evidence seems to show, we are indeed 'being played with', we can learn to play the game and ultimately to manipulate it. We don't even have to take refuge in the unreality of rationalism; we can stay apostates from the Great Conspiracy and still maintain our freedom of choice. We can learn to control the 'controls'; we can create – and dismiss – the illusions of reality.

Dr Morton Schatzman is a psychiatrist living and working in London. In the late 1970s an American woman known simply as Ruth, was referred to him for treatment. Ruth's life was a nightmare; a three-dimensional apparition of her *living* father dogged her everyday life. He had sexually abused her when she was 10 years old and his hallucination made her relive the terror and repugnance. She could see, hear and even smell him, even though she knew he couldn't 'really' be sitting in the living room in London smirking at her, for he was still over in the States. Nobody else saw him but for her he was *there*.

During Ruth's treatment, Schatzman realized that she could hallucinate at will, although the experience left her feeling drained of energy (a point of similarity to seance room phenomena that has not been wasted on psychical researchers). Ruth discovered that only her fear of her father's apparition prevented her from controlling it; experimenting under Schatzman's direction, she learned how to play tricks with her tormentor; treating it scornfully, or refusing to be intimidated by it. On one occasion she merely asked it to pass her a towel when it materialized in her bathroom. Courageously she began to summon it at will, to confront it and control it then, with difficulty, to dismiss it.

Schatzman and his colleagues were amazed at Ruth's ability to create 'doubles' of any people she knew, and although she could not always make them do precisely what she wanted, they went away when she told them to. Clinical tests taken while she obligingly hallucinated showed that Ruth was focusing on something that was 'real' for her. She said her 'people' cast shadows, and were solid to the touch but that their flesh felt colder than that of living beings. Then came the breakthrough: she created a double of her husband that was seen by someone else.

In other times and cultures she would have been branded as a witch, or hailed as a medium, or merely locked away 'for her own good'. But Ruth is not mad and never has been. Schatzman believes that she is extraordinarily creative, able to project her mental images so they appear 'out there', and as real and solid as everyone else. These days she still creates apparitions, but only when she needs company.

BEFORE YOUR VERY EYES

Occultists have long believed that projected thoughtforms can be moulded into creatures that assume enough reality to impinge on the world of flesh and blood. One theory about werewolves is that the hellhounds are embodiments of a sorcerer's desires. Vampires, too, could be created by the will of a powerful magician.

In the late 1960s and early 1970s parapsychologist Dr Jule Eisenbud conducted a series of extraordinary experiments with an alcoholic Chicago bellhop, Ted Serios, who could project images straight on to the emulsion of film in sealed cameras. His 'thoughtographs' were often, despite the inevitable sceptical 'explanation' of fraud, unlike any known photographs of the target locality. It seemed as if they had been taken from a point high in the air, and from a curious angle. The images were also fuzzy with haloes of light and sometimes they were subtly changed from the real thing. The exteriors of buildings, for example, might be changed from smooth stone to a pebble dash effect, or an old facade imposed upon the new.

In recent years, Japanese parapsychologists have produced a great many impressive thoughtographs through their psychic subjects, and Uri Geller has produced some oddities on film, but interestingly, Ruth could not.

T.S. Eliot said: 'Mankind cannot bear too much reality'; but perhaps it becomes more bearable if we can make it do interesting things? The 'reality' of the Great Conspiracy — there's a place for everything and everything must be kept in its place — is in fact an illusion. Life is much more fun than that. One could, for example, create a ghost.

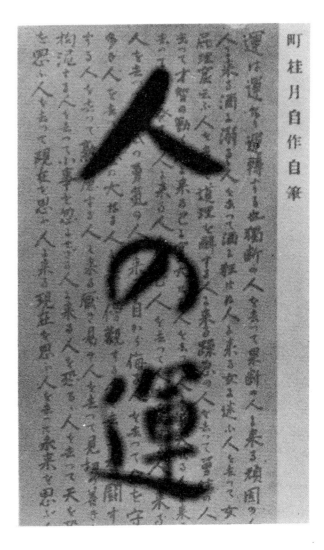

A 'thoughtograph'; the imprint of a purely mental image onto a photographic plate. Although the best-known were produced in the 1960s by a Chicago bellhop, Ted Serios, this is one of many produced by the Japanese psychic Tenshin Takeuchi, during experiments conducted by Dr Fukurai in 1915. Takeuchi managed to produce a whole sentence from a book as well as three letters requested by the psychical researcher. Thoughtographs challenge our ideas about reality itself; if thoughts can be made 'real' enough to impinge on photographic film then our beliefs, which are reinforced thoughts, can surely create all manner of amazing effects such as visions, ghosts or aliens. Is our everyday world merely the product of a consensus of belief?

PHILIP THE PHANTOM PHANTOM

In 1972 a group of members of the Toronto Society for Psychical Research, led by Dr A.R.G. Owen and his wife Iris, began to create the 'ghost' of an entirely fictitious character, whom they called 'Philip'. Before he could make his presence felt every member of the group had to believe in him. His personality and background had to be known to them all, so one member with a flair for romantic fiction wrote his tragic lovelorn history, set in seventeenth-century England, and another member drew his portrait.

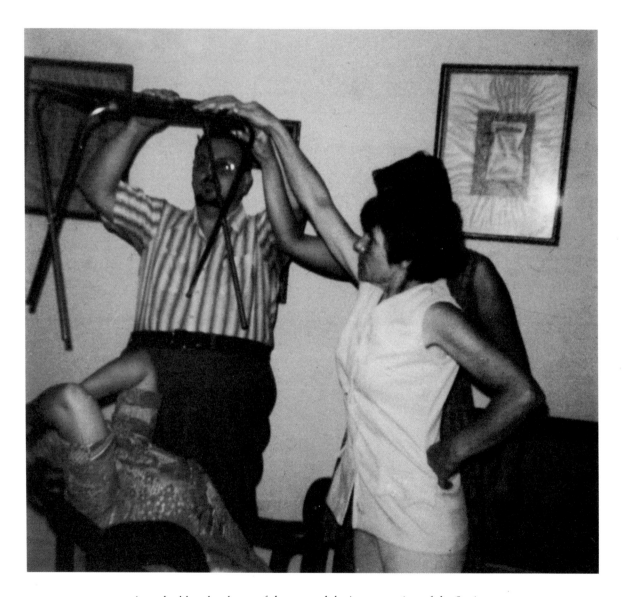

A card table takes leave of the ground during a meeting of the Society for Research on Rapport and Telekinesis (SORRAT) in Missouri. The group met regularly for over twenty years in an atmosphere of belief and encouragement; the phenomena they recorded were spectacular.

Like the meetings of the Society for Research on Rapport and Telekinesis, and Home's seances, they met in a relaxed and jokey atmosphere punctuated with sing-songs. They talked to the table as if it were Philip, resting their hands on it lightly. After months, things began to happen. Philip had arrived.

The table responded to each member's cheery greeting of 'Hello, Philip' by emitting raps under his or her hands. In the classic seance room fashion, 'he' began to answer their questions by rapping out his replies, which always agreed with the details of his history as written by the group, and occasionally

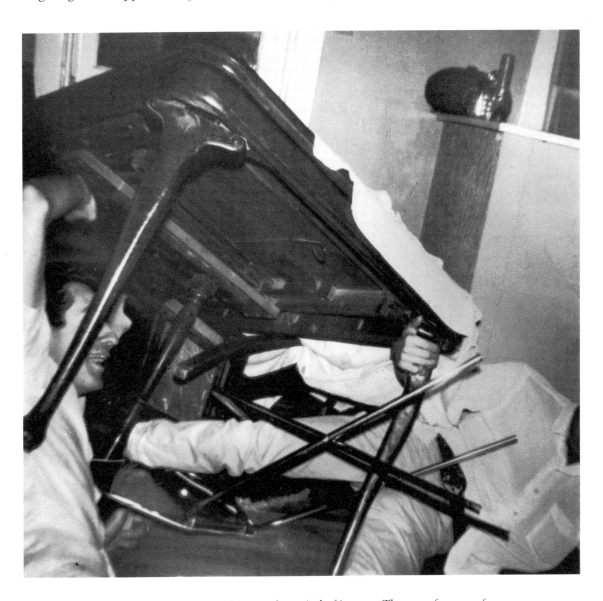

Another SORRAT table reveals a mind of its own. The most famous of all wooden stars, however, was 'Philip' the physical presence of a deliberately-created ghost, a product of the Toronto Society for Psychical Research. Happily cavorting about, 'he' starred in a television programme.

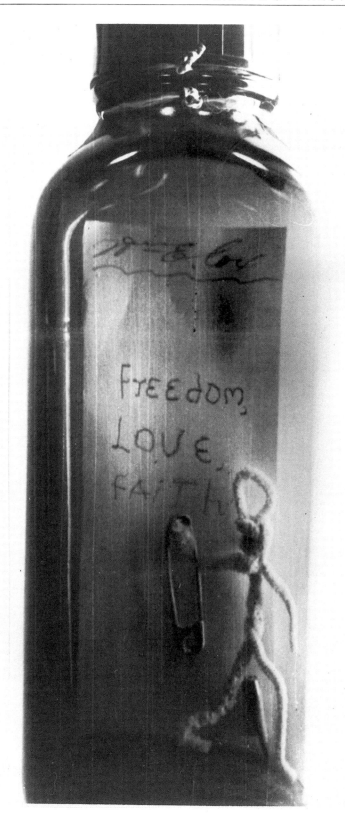

SORRAT's successes crash the 'boggle barrier'. This sealed jar was part of researcher W.E. Cox's experiments on behalf of SORRAT, at the McDonnell Laboratory for Psychical Research in St Louis, Missouri. It contained an open safety pin, a slip of signed paper, a pencil stub and two straight pipe-cleaners. On 24 May 1981, an alleged psychic (not part of SORRAT) was brought in by Cox to try to exert conscious mind over matter on the bottle, which lay on a table across the room. Within the sealed bottle the pencil picked itself up and wrote 'Freedom, Love, Faith', the safety pin closed and the pipe-cleaners formed themselves into a stick man. Although the 'psychic' later confessed himself a fraud, this experiment remained unexplained. It may be that the man's imposture was over-ruled by the power and belief of the group (who at the time believed him to be genuine), or perhaps the Cosmic Joker enjoyed discomforting the fraud by using him to produce genuine phenomena of staggering proportions. In the world of psychical research, the more spectacular the phenomena, the more vicious the attacks from both professional debunkers and fellow researchers. SORRAT has been the butt of a particularly savage campaign, but its members remain serene in the knowledge of what really happened.

he even added to it. Philip proved to be a jolly fellow, joining in their rowdy drinking song by bumping up and down in time to the tune, and he began to behave like a friendly dog – one of his games was to chase people out of the room (on one occasion he got stuck in the doorway). But his finest hour came when he was asked to be a television star.

The group took Philip (the table) to the studios of Toronto City Television in 1974. They sat with him, in case of stage fright perhaps, with the studio audience on the floor, while the presenter sat on the platform with a discussion panel. Philip took to the limelight with a panache that would have put Katie King to shame. He replied to the presenter's hesitant 'Hello, Philip' with a hearty rap, then took off for a tour of inspection, 'walking' by swinging his legs along, like a table might in a Disney cartoon. Then he skipped up the three steps to the platform and proceeded to answer any questions put to him by the panel or the audience by rapping happily.

Like all paranormal phenomena, Philip thrived on belief, and sulked if doubts were expressed. Once a member of the group told him: 'We only made you up, you know,' and the raps abruptly ceased. The group had to take a crash course in building up their belief in him before he would 'perform' again. One is reminded of Peter Pan trying to revive the dying Tinker Bell by asking the audience to 'clap hands if you believe in fairies'. Nobody has let her die yet.

SEEING THE FUNNY SIDE

Are all religious visions, spirit guides, fairies and little green men from Mars actually creations of our own mind, or products of contemporary culture – or are there separate entities 'out there' waiting to take us over? Is it dangerous to cultivate the impossible?

In this illusion-prone world, anything is possible, but it is worth noting that the psychics and sensitives who have survived their visions and visitations seem to have one trait in common: a well-developed sense of humour. Matthew Manning, Uri Geller, Doris Stokes, the Cottingley girls, SORRAT and Philip groups have all shown themselves capable of good, hearty belly laughs. As comedian and psychical researcher Michael Bentine has pointed out, nothing banishes negative forces more effectively than hearty laughter.

Fear and scepticism have been shown time and time again to inhibit the more amusing and useful paranormal phenomena, especially if you actually want them to happen, as in parapsychological investigation. The 'experimenter effect' is the ultimate double bind among researchers: those who believe get the results they want, and those who don't, don't. In other words they get what they expect. If we want more we only have to carry on believing.

The paranormal should be fun.

5

□ CURIOUSER AND CURIOUSER □

THE UNIVERSE BEGAN sixteen billion years ago. We know because apparently we have the technology to find this out, or so the cosmologists tell us. Giant telescopes engineered by scientists with enough letters after their names to stretch from here to the moon, and neat mathematical formulae concocted by men with nothing better to do have, we are told, finally proved that there was no intelligence necessary behind the Big Bang that created all there was, is and ever shall be. God is a redundant concept; rationalism and computers have killed him off – another triumph, as the media machine might say, from the people who brought you carbon- and computer-dating, (which both deal in blind dates.)

But wait. Even to the most abject member of the Great Conspiracy there must be a niggling doubt. Apart from the monumental arrogance involved in attempting to define the history of the universe in our terms and actually claiming to have done so, there seems to be something suspiciously round about that figure of 16 billion. Almost, one might say, unscientific. Why not 15.93 billion or 16.02 billion years ago? Quite a large number of people would believe scientists no matter what they said. After all, 'there is one born every minute' (or is it more precisely every 60.03 seconds?). Some of us are still waiting for the final tally of the number of angels on the head on a pin.

Schoolchildren were once taught, and possibly still are, that the scientific method is based upon observation. If that is true then it is we who are the scientists, we apostates enjoying ourselves enormously in the wilderness with only the odd burning bush to keep us warm. That arch deflator of scientific egos, Charles Fort, dismissed the pomposity of astronomers as being led 'by a cloud of rubbish by day and a pillar of bosh by night...' and that was years before technology had advanced enough to tell us when the universe began.

We are the ones who allow ourselves to observe Newton's apple when it chooses to go up instead of down, the key *untouched* by Uri Geller that bends by itself when he has left the room, the sticky mess that was once a person, and the tennis ball that flies through the mesh of an irreproachable Wimbledon net...we observe anomalies as they happen, and welcome our knowledge of them instead of excluding such leprous data from decent society. They are 'the damned' beloved of Charles Fort, a sage, sly commentator on life on this planet, who is naturally despised by scientists. He has been much quoted throughout this book and it is time he took centre stage.

A MAN FOR ALL SEASONS

Charles Hoy Fort was born in 1874 in Albany, New York and died there in 1932. The son of a sadistic Dutch immigrant he hated authority from an early age and as soon as he could, ran away to hitch-hike around the world in search of putting 'some capital into the bank of experience'. But on returning home he realized that 'one should not scatter one's self upon all life, but center upon some one kind of life and know it thoroughly.' He set out with obsessive thoroughness to read about science. He consumed books, magazines, learned exchanges between professors in the correspondence columns of newspapers and, by the time he was twenty-three, he had made 25,000 notes on the apparent infallibility of science. He burnt them. He then began to amass several thousand more notes, and to write two rather unusual books, entitled *X* and *Y*. The first book

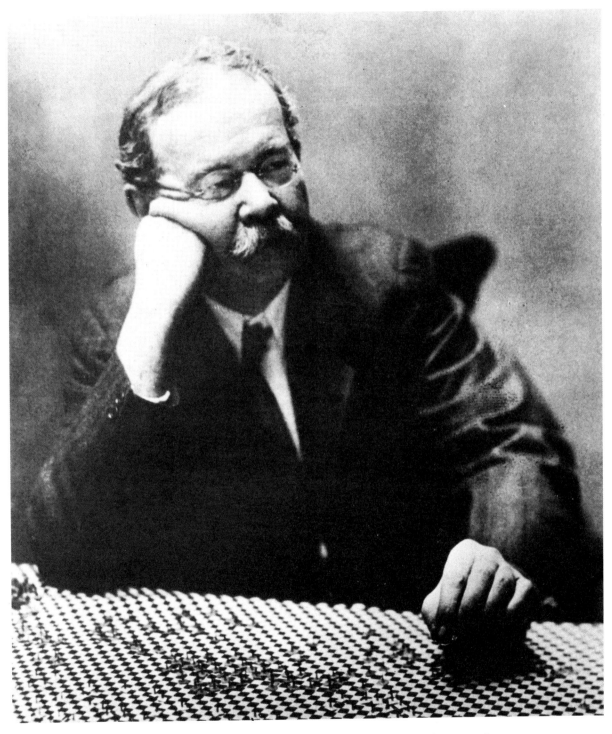

Charles Fort at his 'super chequerboard'. The collector of reports of
anomalous happenings, Fort suggested that Man is at the mercy of a
whimsical Cosmic Joker; that 'we are being played with'.

concerned the idea that earth was a colony of the Martians, and the second that a secret organization lived at the South Pole. On failing to find a publisher he burnt the manuscripts, but if his later style is characteristic no doubt he adhered to the sacred duty of all Wise Fools and court jesters to hide remarkable insights among remorseless facetiousness. As he said, '...as with all clowns, underlying buffoonery is the desire to be taken seriously.'

The death of a relative had left him with a small private income, enough to afford him the freedom to spend his days gorging himself on the riches of the New York Public Library, and occasionally in making pilgrimages across the Atlantic to the British Museum Library. He collected thousands of reports of anomalous happenings from all over the world, and rejoiced in the impossibility of explaining them – and the absurdity of trying to explain them *away*. He wrote to a critic who had accused him, among other crimes, of riotous inconsistency:

> I have pointed out that, though there's nothing wrong with me personally, I am a delusion in super-imagination, and inconsistency must therefore be expected from me – but if I'm so rational as to be aware of my irrationality? Why, then I have glimmers of the awakening and awareness of super-imagination.

Fort loved non-explanations, he knew they were the only sort that survive. 'One measures a circle,' he said, 'beginning anywhere.'

Although he published three other books: *New Lands* (1923), *Lo!* (1931) and *Wild Talents* (1932), it is his first, *The Book of the Damned* (1919), that shows off his uniquely quirky, infuriating and iconoclastic style to perfection. For example, he muses upon our real fate: 'I think we're property...That once upon a time, this earth was No-Man's-Land, that other worlds explored and colonized here, and fought among themselves for possession, but now it's owned by something, all others warned off.'

His style was to assault the reader with weird facts and weirder theories to account for them; sometimes defiant, sometimes apparently contradictory and often deliberately hilarious. He took a firm stand about science:

> Our antagonism is not to Science, but to the attitude of the sciences that they have finally realized; or belief, instead of acceptance; to the insufficiency, which, as we have seen over, amount to paltriness and puerility of scientific dogmas and standards. Or, if several persons start out to Chicago, and get to Buffalo, and one be under the delusion that Buffalo is Chicago, that one will be resistance to the progress of the others.

Critics did not know what to make of *The Book of the Damned*. It is not the easiest of reading; teasing and challenging, buffeting and blinding with science, pseudo-science and theories that, wild as they may seem, are disturbingly compelling.

It was based on an enormous collection of 'anomalistics'; reports of mysterious falls of fish, stones, black and red rains, and bizarre Chinese seals that fell on Ireland. (As Fort said: 'Not the things with the big wistful eyes that lie on ice, and that are taught to balance objects on their noses – but inscribed stamps, with which to make impressions.')

Taken from *The Proceedings of the Royal Irish Academy* and *Chambers' Journal* for 1852, the data seem cynic-proof. Small cube-shaped seals bearing raised animals and Chinese inscriptions were found in almost every Irish county. About sixty were reported and presumably many more remained unnoticed or were, in the nature of unconsidered trifles, pocketed without a word. Fort noted: 'It is the astonishing scattering of them, over field and forest, that has hushed the explainers', and one Dr Frazer wrote: 'The invariable story of their find is what we might expect if they had been accidentally dropped...' But Fort added slyly: '...one of these Chinese seals was found in the bed of the River Boyne, near Clonard, Meath, when workmen were raising gravel. That one, at least, had been dropped there.'

'THIS IS A VICE WE'RE WRITING'

Elsewhere in this monumental and argumentative work he remarks: 'I think this is a vice we're writing. I recommend it to those who have hankered for a new sin'.

Fort was particularly taken with the many accounts of anomalous falls of fish and frogs that peppered his researches. Most of these pisces from heaven fell after or during heavy rain, thus giving rise to rationalist explanations that they have been scooped up in one place by the elements and dropped in another. Minnows and sticklebacks fell on the astonished residents of Mountain Ash, Glamorganshire, Wales in February 1859, while a shower of small *white* frogs fell on the startled people of Birmingham. 'Were there some special froggy place near Europe,' wrote Fort, '... the scientific explanation would of course be that all small frogs falling from the sky in Europe come from the centre of frogeity.'

Frogs have a penchant for abrupt departures. I had a tank of adolescent frogs once, of which I was very proud, watching their first tentative hops much as any mother coos over her toddler's attempts to walk. One night I checked that none of them could jump higher than halfway up the side of the tank, then went to bed, sad that I would soon have to take them to a pond I knew (where all my frogs went eventually). But perhaps they went by themselves; next morning not one of the tiny froglets remained. They were not hiding under the rocks nor squashed on the floor, nor were any tiny corpses found rotting or dried anywhere in the flat. They had been taken in the night, perhaps to the 'centre of frogeity', awaiting a final plunge on to the head of an innocent passerby in Paris, Manchester or Little Rock, Arkansas.

Fort coined the term 'teleportation' to describe the mysterious process that takes up living beings and objects from one place and deposits them elsewhere, not necessarily in mint condition. In November 1888 the bodies of two local men were found among some trees in Birmingham, Alabama. They had been brutally murdered – as had a complete stranger whose battered body was found with them. No one remembered seeing him in the area and he was never identified. In the 1920s the body of a man 'of superior class' (judging only by his smooth skin and manicured hands, for he was naked) was found in a ploughed field near Petersfield, Hampshire. He had died from exposure only a mile or so from the nearest house. His clothes were nowhere to be found and he was never identified. At Chillerton, Isle of Wight, a farmer locked away his twelve calves for the night; next morning there were thirteen. The interloper was a very young white calf without any identifying mark. A large goldfish disappeared from a pond and fourteen small ones appeared in its place...

Fort proposed that teleportation had once been a much more powerful force, distributing whole beings, and sometimes their component parts, around the inhabitable planets, but the demand has dwindled and '...the cosmic humour of it all – that the force that once heaped the peaks of the Rocky Mountains now slings pebbles at a couple of farmers near Trenton, New Jersey.'

He saw all the 'damned data' of psychic phenomena as being essentially the same, differing only as the fashion differs. Thus if an object disappears from a seance room it is deemed the work of spirits and if it disappears from the home of a UFO contactee it has been removed by aliens. (If it disappears from the home of a scientist then it was probably never there in the first place.) But all this appearing and disappearing is really due to the action of a sort of giant magnet, the ancient teleportive force, which now perhaps is making only random sorties upon the stocks of people and things on earth. This force moves in mysterious ways.

In 1666 the shower of fish that fell in Kent fell in one particular field and in Calcutta in September 1839 fish fell *in a straight line*, 'not more than one cubit in breadth', rather as if poured down an invisible tube. Dead and dried fish fell in Futtepoor and Allahabad in India in the 1830s, and in 1896 a carp fell on Essen, Germany, that was preserved in a block of ice. If there are 'more things in Heaven and Earth than are dreamt of...' then they keep falling on us without warning.

Fort unearthed reports of falls of blood and decomposing organic matter, lumps of jelly, toads, periwinkles, cinders, oily substances, stones (large, small and curiously inscribed), and indeed most things that cannot possibly lurk in our skies waiting to fall on us. They can and they do.

As Fort said in *Lo!*:

> I have collected 294 records of showers of living things. Have I? Well, there's no accounting for the freaks of industry. It is the profound conviction of most of us that there never has been a shower of living things. But some of us have, at least in an elementary way, been educated by surprises out of much that we are 'absolutely sure of', and are suspicious of a thought, simply because it is a profound conviction.

'THERE IN THE FIRST PLACE'

Of course these 'damned' data must be explained away; the Cosmic Litterlout must be ignored. The rationalists are fond of crowing: 'they [anomalous objects fallen from the skies] must have been there in the first place', or if pressed very hard to do better, then the 'experts' fall over themselves to find the most facile explanation for the strange cargoes that shower on us. In 1980 a shower of little green frogs fell on Athens, Greece; experts talked loosely of whirlwinds. None had been reported locally, and it would be a strange whirlwind indeed that selects only fish or frogs from the assorted debris it must suck up in its travels. Besides, whirlwinds move with a determined swiftness: in 1918 the Tyneside town of Sunderland was pelted with sand eels for ten minutes.

The minnows and sticklebacks that splattered Mountain Ash were mostly alive when they hit the ground. One even survived the journey to Dr Gray of the British Museum who lost no time in declaring: 'On reading the evidence, it seems to me most probably a practical joke that one of Mr Nixon's employees had thrown a pailful of water upon another who had thought fish in it had fallen from the sky...' (In *The Book of the Damned* Fort remarks: 'My own notion is that it is very unsportsmanlike ever to mention fraud. Accept anything. Then explain it your way.')

But these fish had fallen over a very wide area, once. Then, ten minutes later, fish fell again over precisely the same long, narrow strip of Welsh land. If it were a hoax, the Joker was not a local lad. Fort suggests 'That the bottom of a super-geographical pond had dropped out.' Even this theory fits the facts rather better than a fictitious whirlwind.

Fort said:

> I think of a region somewhere above this earth's surface in which gravitation is inoperative... I think that things raised from this earth's surface to that region have been held there until shaken down by storms – the Super-Sargasso Sea. Derelicts, rubbish, old cargoes from inter-planetary wrecks; things cast out into what is called space by convulsions of other planets, things from the times of the Alexanders, Caesars and Napoleons of Mars and Jupiter and Neptune...horses and barns and elephants and flies and dodoes, moas and pterodactyls...fishes dried and hard, there a short time: others there long enough to putrefy.

Sometimes objects seem to be deliberately aimed at specific people by the Cosmic Joker with his mighty catapult. John Michell notes in his *Phenomena: a Book of Wonders* (1977) that one A.D. Bajkov, an ichthyologist, was chosen to be pelted with fish on 22 April 1949, and on 2 April 1973 Dr Richard Griffiths, a Manchester meteorologist, was nearly hit by a lump of ice that fell at his feet. Upon examination it proved to be of unknown origin. In December 1974 a school in Berkshire, England

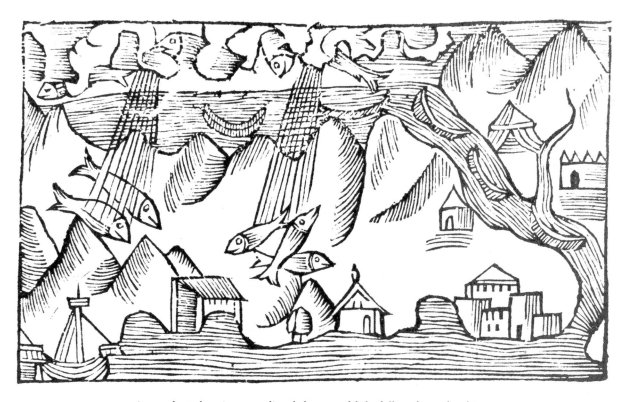

A woodcut showing a medieval shower of fish, falling from the skies.
Fishfalls are one of a huge number of 'Fortean' phenomena that defy
rational explanation and seem to be the work of some ultra-terrestrials
who, judging by the sheer volume and variety of things dumped on us,
must be cosmic litterlouts. Attempts at prosaic explanations are often, as
Fort's researches showed, sillier than the events themselves.

was repeatedly bombarded by eggs, apparently falling from a great height. The school was called Keep Hatch.

HOLDING THE LOOKING GLASS UP TO NATURE

We are more truly creative than we think – Ruth's hallucinations and Philip the phantom phantom (Chapter 4) pose fascinating questions about the role of imagination in making subjective reality become objective, sending it 'out there' rather than locked in our minds. The world of the arts in particular provides the Joker with a storyline, in the classic Fortean role reversal where life appears to imitate art

and not as most people fondly suppose, vice versa.

The science writer Arthur Koestler was particularly fascinated by spectacular coincidences, where each component dovetails so neatly with the others that a positive pattern seems to emerge. He collated hundreds of cases of what psychologist Carl Gustav Jung called 'synchronicity', or an 'acausal connecting principle' – the irresistible linking of people and events through no known agency. One such case was that of London writer Pearl Binder, who, together with friends George and Olive Ordish amused themselves by 'planning a joint satirical novel' in the autumn of 1966, which was published six years later under the title *Ladies Only*:

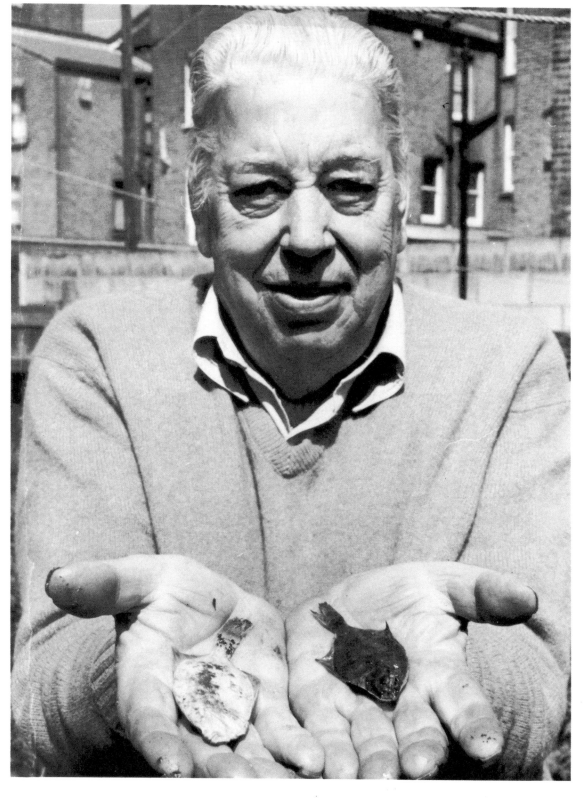

Our idea was then in its earliest stages, the plot still vague, and the characters not even formulated. On the spur of the moment I suggested, 'Why shouldn't it be in the future, when the population explosion will have made London almost uninhabitable? There would be camps set up in Hyde Park for the homeless. Let's have a refugee professor camping out there.' 'Viennese,' put in Mr Ordish, 'a broken-down old savant.' 'All goulash and sentiment,' added Mrs Ordish, 'with one of those unpronounceable Hungarian-sounding names...Nadoly...Horvath-Nadoly.' And we went on to think of other characters. A couple of days later we were astounded to read a news item in the morning press reporting that a homeless foreign old man had been found by police wandering alone at night in Hyde Park. He gave his name as Horvath-Nadoly.

Pearl Binder added: 'we felt we had invented this tramp, and in the process brought him to life, and a pretty awful life.' Had the derelict with the impossible name been teleported from a plane that only exists when we trigger it into being with certain words? ('In the beginning was the word...') Had the writers' intense – and joint – search for a ridiculous name directed them to the appropriate section of some vast paranormal set of yellow pages?

Mr Ron Langton showing just some of the dozen flounders and smelts that fell on his East London home on 28 May 1984. Sometimes tiny areas are singled out to be dumped on repeatedly, as was one long, narrow strip of Welsh land in 1859 when *live* minnows and sticklebacks fell out of a clear sky twice in ten minutes. Dried fish fell in India, and frogs have fallen everywhere. Fort, tongue-in-cheek as ever, suggested that there may be a 'centre of frogeity' over Europe, whence fall the frogs. He may even have been right; no one else has managed satisfactorily to explain the phenomena. 'Experts' commonly blame rogue whirlwinds for picking up the creatures in one place and dropping them elsewhere – but in that case what happens to the other debris?

ALL THE WORLD'S A STAGE

Anomaly researchers have noted that entertainers and writers seem to attract more synchronistic happenings than most other people. Perhaps it is their business of creating and acting out fictional lives that provokes a challenge to the Joker. Perrott Phillips in *The Unexplained* tells a story involving both an actor and a writer:

The British actor Anthony Hopkins was delighted to hear he had landed a leading role in a film based on the book *The Girl From Petrovka* by George Feifer. A few days after signing the contract, Hopkins travelled to London to buy a copy of the book. He tried several bookshops, but there wasn't one to be had. Waiting at Leicester Square underground for his train home, he noticed a book lying apparently discarded on a bench. Incredibly, it was *The Girl from Petrovka*. That in itself would have been coincidence enough but in fact it was merely the beginning of an extraordinary chain of events. Two years later, in the middle of filming in Vienna, Hopkins was visited by George Feifer, the author. Feifer mentioned that he did not have a copy of his own book. He had lent the last one – containing his own annotations – to a friend who had lost it somewhere in London. With mounting astonishment, Hopkins handed Feifer the book he had found: 'Is this the one?' he asked, 'with the notes scribbled in the margins?' It was the same book.

Some actors and their associates are condemned to suffer a similar fate to those of the characters they have portrayed. The opera singer Marie Collier was cheerfully discussing her future career with her manager when she opened a window and inexplicably fell. She was killed instantly. Her last part had been that of Tosca, who leaps to her death.

In 1979 Lesley and Jonathan Heele unwittingly took over the tragedy of the parents in the film *Don't Look Now* (1973), played by Julie Christie and Donald Sutherland, when they were living in Miss Christie's farmhouse in Wales. The film actress was about to leave after a short visit when Lesley discovered her toddler's body floating in a shallow pond – the fate of the child in the film.

The *Daily Mail* of 26 June 1985 (and later the *Fortean Times*) notes: 'The actor originally hired to play John Lennon in the recent BBC TV dramatization, "A Journey in the Life", was fired when Lennon's wife, Yoko, discovered that he bore the same name as the Beatle's assassin, Mark Chapman. Actor Chapman had changed his name to Lindsay in the year Lennon was killed.'

A LITTLE KNOWLEDGE...

Sometimes the revelation of unconscious foreknowledge can land one in trouble with the authorities, as these two examples show:

One of the best kept secrets of the Second World War was the planned Allied Invasion of Europe in June 1944. Each component of the campaign's jigsaw was referred to only by codewords: the operation itself was OVERLORD, the naval attack was to be known as NEPTUNE, the artificial harbours used in the landing were MULBERRY and the Normandy beaches where the Allies were to land were called UTAH and OMAHA.

British Intelligence chiefs were appalled to discover that, in the month before D-Day, all these codewords featured as the answer to clues in the *The Daily Telegraph* crossword:

- Seventeen across: 'One of the U.S.', four letters.
- Eleven across: 'This bush is a centre of nursery revolution', eight letters.
- Three down: 'Red Indian on the Missouri', five letters.
- Thirteen down: 'Britannia and he hold to the same thing', seven letters.
- Eleven across: 'But some big-wig like this has stolen some of it at times', eight letters.

The final answer was OVERLORD itself, just four days before 6 June. The authorities swooped on the Fleet Street office of that august newspaper, expecting to find a Nazi master spy menacing its genteel atmosphere redolent of old school tie and cricket scores. But the newspaper's crossword genius was the least likely friend of the Third Reich imaginable – Leonard Dawe, a schoolmaster who had compiled crosswords for 20 years. He was subjected to intense interrogation but finally it had to be admitted that Mr Dawe was innocent. It was a coincidence.

One may imagine that Leonard Dawe's creative process somehow plucked the codewords from the air – they 'just came to him' perhaps.

The Joker would find the incongruity of harmless Mr Dawe's interrogation, while the whole Allied war machine believes itself betrayed by him, highly amusing. But as it happened, Hitler did not take the *The Daily Telegraph* anyway.

Alan Vaughan in his *Incredible Coincidence* (1978) tells the sinister tale of the pornographic novel that foretold 'with stunning accuracy the events of the Patricia Hearst kidnapping of 1974.' *Black Abductor* by Harrison James (real name James Rusk) was first published in 1972; Vaughan reveals how the novel foretold the Hearst case in almost every detail:

A young college student named Patricia, daughter of a wealthy and prominent right-wing figure, is kidnapped near the campus while she is with her boyfriend, who is severely beaten. The kidnappers, led by an angry young black man, are members of a terrorist revolutionary group. At first, the girl is an unwilling captive but later adopts the ideology and joins the group. They send Polaroid pictures of her to her father, along with messages, in what is termed America's 'first political kidnapping'. The fictional abductors predict that they will ultimately be surrounded by the police, tear-gassed, and killed.

About four weeks after the Hearst kidnapping, Rusk was visited by the FBI and shown pictures of the SLA group that had kidnapped her. Evidently, after learning of the book, the FBI suspected that Rusk had either been in on the planning of the kidnapping or that the SLA had gotten the idea from reading his book. In other words the FBI assumed there must be a causal connection between the book and the event. But then the FBI doesn't know about unconscious foreknowledge.

Despite a few uncomfortable days of being grilled by the FBI, author 'Harrison James' came out of this remarkable coincidence rather well: the book was reissued under the title *Abduction: Fiction Before Fact* and proved, for him at least, a novel way to make crime pay.

An early-twentieth-century theory to account for coincidence was Dr Paul Kammerer's 'law of seriality', first published in his native German in 1919. Seriality, he believed, 'is the umbilical cord that connects thought, feeling, science and art with the womb of the universe which gave birth to them'. Everything is part of everything else, but people and events with something particular in common – names or dates – tend to cluster together.

Jung's idea of 'synchronicity' embraced the concept of 'two or more causally unrelated events which have the same or similar meaning' seeking each other out to make a meaningful coincidence. He also said: 'synchronicity suggests that there is an interconnection or unity of causally unrelated events, and thus

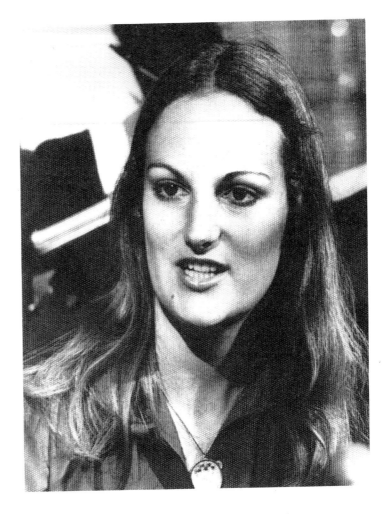

Patricia Hearst, kidnap victim turned terrorist. The dramatic story of her conversion was found to tally in every detail with a fictional story by James Rusk, *Black Abductor*, written before the event. Not unnaturally the FBI seized Rusk and interrogated him, believing him to have had prior knowledge of the kidnapping. In the end, however, they let him go. This was just another story of art, instead of imitating life, behaving contrariwise. Can the creative imagination actually cause events to happen, providing, as it were, the plot and storyline for the Cosmic Joker to use against us? Perhaps it is literally true that: 'All the world's a stage, and all the men and women merely players...'

postulates a unitary aspect of being.' As Alan Vaughan says, 'This is not easy to see.'

The writer who has done the most to popularize the mysteries of coincidence was undoubtedly Arthur Koestler, whose books *The Roots of Coincidence* (1972) and *The Challenge of Chance* (1974), written with Alister Hardy and Robert Harvie, postulate a universe constantly striving to impose order and meaning on itself.

The 'lexilinking', the striking verbal connections that recur time and time again in every coincidence file, is as good a way as any other to bring otherwise unconnected people together in an event that temporarily makes some sort of sense of the world.

In 1985 John Stott crashed his car, witnessed by one Bernard Stott. The case was investigated by WPC Tina Stott and booked by desk sergeant Walter Stott. Of course it would still have been remarkable had they all shared the surname Smith or Jones.

The quite ordinary names Lincoln and Kennedy were linked across time in tragic synchronicity that is so horribly deft in all its details it seems to have been a *danse macabre* staged by some monstrous choreographer:

- Both Presidents Lincoln and Kennedy were concerned with civil rights.
- Lincoln was elected president in 1860; Kennedy in 1960.
- Both were slain on a Friday and in the presence of their wives.
- Both were shot from behind and in the head.
- Their successors, both named Johnson, were Southern Democrats, and both were in the Senate.
- Andrew Johnson was born in 1808 and Lyndon Johnson in 1908.
- The assassins, John Wilkes Booth and Lee Harvey Oswald were born in 1839 and 1939 respectively.
- Booth and Oswald were southerners favouring unpopular ideas.
- Both presidents had children die while they lived in the White House.

- Lincoln's secretary, whose name was Kennedy, advised him not to go to the theatre.
- Kennedy's secretary, whose name was Lincoln, advised him not to go to Dallas.
- Booth shot Lincoln in a theatre and ran to a warehouse.
- Oswald shot Kennedy from a warehouse and ran to a theatre.
- The names Lincoln and Kennedy each contain seven letters.
- The names John Wilkes Booth and Lee Harvey Oswald contain fifteen letters.
- The names Andrew Johnson and Lyndon Johnson each contain thirteen letters.
- Both assassins were killed before being brought to trial.

At this point a cold chill blows around the concept of freewill.

But consider this recent case of lexilinking across time, which may be taken as a validation of prophecy on a grand scale – up to a point. In April 1986 the name of an obscure Soviet town was on everyone's lips: Chernobyl. Those familiar with the Book of Revelations will know that the phoney phase of doom and gloom is over and that the truly nasty business of the latter days is settling in, with the Four Horsemen of the Apocalypse saddling up in the wings. For Chernobyl means wormwood in Ukrainian and, according to the Bible's most extravagant pessimist, St John of Patmos (*Revelations* Chapter 8; 10–11):

And the third angel sounded, and there fell a great star from heaven, burning as it were a lamp and fell upon the third part of the rivers, and upon the fountains of the waters.

And the name of the star is called Wormwood; and the third part of the waters became wormwood: and many died of the waters, because they were made bitter.

Fortean Times (issue 47) carried notes on further connections between the name of the Ukrainian town and doom and disaster. P. J. Edmonds of West Sussex wrote to *The Daily Telegraph*: 'Chernobyl may also be translated as 'a black event', while the Fortean commentator adds that 'Chernobog' was a 'chthonian Lord of Death, a "black sun beneath the Earth" in opposition to the heavenly white sun.'

It all seems chillingly apposite, considering the terror in which the world watched as 'Melt Down' approached, threatening to poison the water supplies as well as shroud the atmosphere in creeping death. *But it did not happen.* Melt Down was avoided, the waters were not poisoned. Perhaps, after all, prophecies of the earth's fate are greatly exaggerated. But it was a near thing.

□

As luck would have it...

□

Alan Vaughan believes that:

Consciousness creates space, time and matter ...by means of chance, but at the most fundamental subatomic (quantum) level of reality and at the level of our everyday lives...ordinary cause and effect vanish, to be replaced by probabilities. Which probability is realised depends on the observing consciousness. Psychic phenomena and meaningful coincidence are the very demonstration that consciousness lies outside space and time – and indeed creates them – as it creates our lives.

Vaughan believes that the greater our need, the more likely helpful coincidences are to happen. Most people have at least one experience of Fate stepping in, at the last minute, to alleviate the throes of a crisis. The eight-stone mother suddenly finds the strength to lift the family car off her child (there are many such recorded cases); or dolphins appear 'from nowhere' and chase off the marauding sharks; the insurance man who went to the wrong house notices that gas leak; after months of searching, the perfect house turns up, casually mentioned by a fellow guest at a dinner party you nearly didn't attend.

Perhaps this 'luck' is the sudden surfacing of our own creativity, activated through the pressure of great need, although the chain of cause and effect may be immensely complex, and reach over time and space in a way that is not always easy to trace back.

I have had many experiences of eleventh-hour relief, and while it might be tempting the Joker too much to come to rely on them, they have made me positively Micawberish in my belief that 'something will turn up'. One incident had both immediate and long-term benefits for me:

Part of my duties as Deputy Editor of the weekly publication *The Unexplained* was to plan and commission future articles, and as the original 120-week run was to be extended, finding subjects and authors to fill five or six articles each week became increasingly difficult. One week absolute disaster struck; one article simply did not turn up; we had that publisher's nightmare, six blank pages in an issue of twenty. None of our future articles could be brought forward, and the deadline for that particular issue was only a day away.

In despair I turned to the mail; there on the top was an envelope containing an unsolicited article by Dr A.G. Khan, telling the story of his daughter Durdana's experiences in the spirit while her body was, for a few minutes, clinically dead. Not only was it a fascinating and moving story, but it was so beautifully written it barely needed a touch of the proverbial blue pencil; and as a bonus Dr Khan had enclosed some of Durdana's paintings of the place she visited when she was 'dead'. (A recurring nightmare for a highly illustrated publication like *The Unexplained* was the Unillustratable Monster of an article.) But suddenly, in one bolt from the blue, we had everything and when typed out to the measure it even fitted the number of pages we so desperately needed to the line.

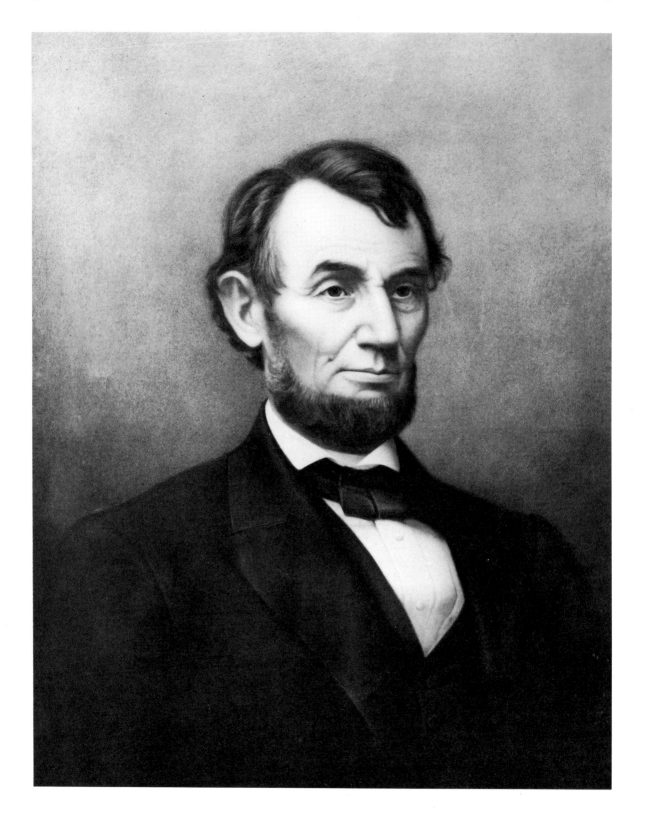

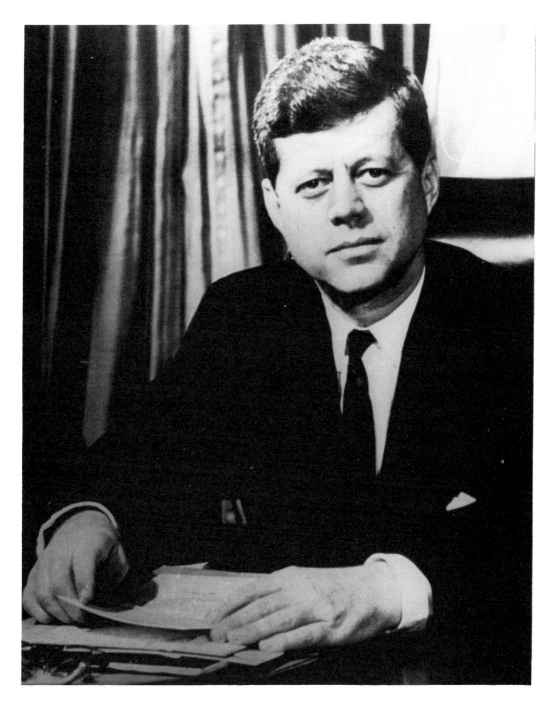

Some coincidences are so striking and are so horrifying that they seem to have been engineered by some malign power for its own amusement. The lives, and more particularly the deaths, of Presidents Lincoln and Kennedy reveal such black humour at work. At least seventeen remarkable links between them have been discovered, including the facts that Lincoln had a secretary called Kennedy, and Kennedy had one called Lincoln; Lincoln was elected in 1860 and Kennedy in 1960; they were both slain on a Friday by assassins whose names each contained fifteen letters and who were born in 1839 and 1939 respectively.

This godsend had yet one more bonus for me personally. At that time my father was very ill with the cancer that was to kill him. Durdana's extraordinary story touched off, for him, a profound sense of hope in an afterlife that traditional platitudes had failed to inspire. It was as if the Khans of far-off Pakistan and the Picknetts of Yorkshire had been compelled to find each other, literally over a matter of life and death. And I had a deadline to meet, after all.

Yet how can I possibly apply the 'needs-must' theory to this coincidence? Surely my rising sense of panic as I sat at my desk, and my father's even greater panic as he lay in his bed, could hardly reach back a few days to inspire Dr Khan to write out the story, and prompt him to type it to precisely the right number of words we needed, and then send it to the office by the last possible post before my deadline? And before that, what prompted him to buy his first copy of the magazine, read it and decide he would like *us* to hear Durdana's tale? What life-giving coincidences for the future of how many lives are we all setting in motion through the simplest of our actions *now*? But although it is an enormously difficult concept to grasp, time is not necessarily an orderly progression, but can run in all directions, fizzing as it goes with the unruly sparks that are our thoughts; pure elemental, creative energy.

MINDS OF THEIR OWN?

Even parapsychologists, who usually confuse labels with explanations, acknowledge a version of the Micawber syndrome of eleventh-hour salvation. They call it Psi-Mediated Instrumental Response (PMIR), the 'instruments' thus referred to being machines, those infuriating lumps of plastic and metal that the ignorant call inanimate. *Nothing* is inanimate.

Research shows an enormous number of cases where machines have inexplicably stalled or broken down in response to some emergency *in our immediate future*, such as the normally reliable invalid car that stalled at a green light on a busy road, to the great inconvenience and embarrassment of the driver. But had it leapt into life and obediently crossed the road it would have met head-on with a runaway truck. When the danger was over, the car started without a whimper. Less dramatically, a teacher's motor mower regularly breaks down as soon as he begins his summer vacation – out of sympathy, perhaps. He hates mowing.

We may need to find a piece of information in a hurry; we pick up a book at random and the 'library angel' obligingly opens it at the relevant page. Or we need to talk to someone and out of the blue *they* telephone *us*. Problems seek solutions, questions provoke answers. Mankind is greatly and uniquely gifted in possessing such wide-ranging creative abilities on all levels of being and that can affect not only today and tomorrow but yesterday too.

Of course not everyone is 'lucky' enough to own a precognitive car or a co-operative motor mower; accidents do happen and chores have to be done (no excuses). But if links can be forged between our minds and our machinery there is no reason – theoretically at least – why you and I can't learn how to harmonize with the objects we think we own. Perhaps we will learn how to *train* our belongings to have some self-respect instead of exhibiting only two modes of behaviour; sulking or flying into terrible 'poltergeist' rages. There must be moderation for tables and chairs as well as their owners.

PIGS MIGHT FLY

The Conspirators are afraid. Deadly afraid. After all, if one rebel tennis ball set a precedent by skimming through the mesh of a net then this could be the end of Wimbledon as we know it. Why should the heresy stop with playthings? If people allow themselves to believe in what is clearly impossible, then who knows? Whole mountains might move.

The Conspirators are afraid of us, and fear

is the weapon they wield. Civilisation is a rather grey labour camp surrounded by the barbed wire of terror, thanks to them. Terror about life, terror about death – and now terror about tennis balls. We fear attack by muggers, viruses, tax demands, bombs – and now falls of dried halibut. We fear the living and the dead. We suffer from *phobiaphobia* (the fear of phobias). But terror, we are taught, is infinitely preferable to its lack, for it keeps things in their place and fear inhibits, so it frightens off the impossible. The circle is complete.

The Conspirators tell us that a belief in mind over matter, or the power to heal without drugs, or in the survival of bodily death will plunge us into further terror – the Dark Ages of superstition. But we must remember that these same guardians of civilisation gave their official approval to the idea of Black Holes. One might as well believe in the Kingdom of Heaven, a much jollier concept – and you don't even have to be a grown-up to get in. 'Be ye as a little child...' ran the good advice on the entry form. We all know that kids have more fun: school's out.

The greatest gift of childhood is imagination, which adults seek to devalue by prefixing with the word 'only'. We have seen, however, that imagination is the stuff of which reality is made. Ruth can create solid hallucinations by manipulating her imagination; Philip was a product of a group's imagination; thoughts can be caught on film. We talk of Uri Geller's psychokinetic powers 'capturing our imagination' when we should be talking of his freeing it, so we can induce similar feats. Just imagine...and nothing is impossible.

Imagine a world where telepathy made telephones and mail obsolete (perhaps one could send celebratory thoughtograms for special occasions?); where the mind monitors its hypersensitive relationship with the body and the spirit, and quashes disharmony before it produces a dis-ease; where loved ones past and present could be summoned up in reassuringly solid form for a cup of tea and a chat; where famine is unknown because crops like us enough to proliferate, even on stony ground (and there's always the nightly falls of manna to fall back on); a world where nothing is impossible. In fact it is this world, now, given the benefit of the doubt.

We could do worse than emulate Lewis Carroll's White Queen and believe 'six impossible things before breakfast', in the sure knowledge that they will have happened to someone somewhere in the world well before lunch.

Yes, in a farmyard in the Urals or on a refuse dump in Calcutta, a small porcine creature is unfurling its wings...

▫ INDEX ▫

ACKNOWLEDGEMENTS

With thanks to: Hilary Evans for pictures on pages 15, 18, 24, 41, 45, 49, 67, 85, 91, 93, 98 (Mary Evans Picture Library); 28, 53 (Mary Evans/Harry Price Coll., Univ. of London); 34, 35, 47 (Mary Evans/Society for Psychical Research); 38, 42 (Mary Evans/Psychic News).

Janet and Colin Bord for pictures on pages 58, 60, 65, 72, 73, 80, 82, 83, 101, 102, 103, 104, 111 (Fortean Picture Library); 107 (Aaron Sussman/Fortean Picture Library). Joe Cooper for pictures on pages 88, 89.

The *Newham Recorder* for picture on page 112.

Guy Lyon Playfair for pictures on pages 30, 51.

Topham Picture Library for pictures on pages 115, 118, 119.

FURTHER READING

There are dozens of excellent books on all aspects of the paranormal. Here is a list of suggested titles that may whet your appetite:

Bentine, Michael *Doors of the Mind* (Panther, 1985)

Bord, Janet and Colin *Modern Mysteries of Britain* (Grafton Books, 1987)

Brookesmith, Peter (ed) *Mysteries of the Church*; *Strange Talents*; *When the Impossible Happens* (Orbis, 1984). These are compilations of articles taken from *The Unexplained* (Orbis, 1980–83).

Cade, Maxwell and Delphine Davis *The Taming of the Thunderbolts* (Abelard-Scuman, 1969)

Cooper, Joe *The Mystery of Telepathy* (Constable, 1982)

Crookes, William *Researches in the Phenomena of Spiritualism* (J. Burns, 1874)

David-Neel, Alexandra *Magic and Mystery in Tibet* (University Books (New York), 1965)

Doyle, Arthur Conan *The Coming of the Fairies* (Hodder and Stoughton, 1922)

Eisenbud, Jule *The World of Ted Serios* (Cape, 1968)

Evans, Hilary *Intrusions* (Routledge & Kegan Paul, 1982); *Visions. Apparitions. Alien Visitors.* (Aquarian Press, 1984)

Fort, Charles *The Complete Books of Charles Fort* (Dover, 1974)

Gaddis, Vincent *Mysterious Fires and Lights* (Dell (New York), 1968)

Gardner, Edward L. *Fairies* (TPH, 1922)

Geller, Uri and Playfair, Guy Lyon *The Geller Effect* (Cape, 1986)

Hall, Trevor H. *The Spiritualists* (Duckworth, 1962); *The Enigma of Daniel Home?* Prometheus Books (Buffalo) 1984)

Harrison, Michael *Fire From Heaven* (Pan, 1977)

Haynes, Renée *The Society for Psychical Research 1882–1982 A history* (Macdonald, 1982)

Home, Daniel Dunglas *Lights and Shadows of Spiritualism* (Virtue, 1877)

Inglis, Brian *Natural and Supernatural* (Abacus, 1977); *Science and Parascience* (Cape, 1984); *The Paranormal: an Encyclopedia of Psychic Phenomena* (Cape, 1985); *The Hidden Power* (Cape, 1986)

Keel, John A. *UFOs: Operation Trojan Horse* (Sphere Abacus, 1973)

Koestler, Arthur *The Roots of Coincidence* (Hutchinson, 1972)

McClure, Kevin *The Evidence for Visions of the Blessed Virgin Mary* (Aquarian Press, 1983)

Manning, Matthew *The Link* (Corgi, 1975)

Michell, John and Rickard, J.M. *Phenomena: a book of wonders* Thames and Hudson, 1977)

Playfair, Guy Lyon *This House is Haunted* (Sphere, 1980)

Randles, Jenny *Beyond Explanation?* (Hale, 1985)

Richards, John Thomas *SORRAT: a History of the Neihardt Psychokinesis Experiments 1961–1981* (Scarecrow Press, 1982)

Roll, W.G. *The Poltergeist* (Star Books, 1976)

Schatzman, Morton *The Story of Ruth* (Duckworth, 1980)

Sladek, John *The New Apocrypha* (Granada, 1978)

Stokes, Doris *A Host of Voices* (Futura, 1984)

Thurston, Herbert J. *The Physical Phenomena of Mysticism* (Burns Oates, 1952); *Ghosts and Poltergeists* (Burns Oates, 1953)

Vaughan, Alan *Incredible Coincidence* (Corgi, 1981)

Wilson, Colin *Poltergeist!* (NEL, 1981)

SOME USEFUL ADDRESSES

ASSAP (Association for the Scientific Study of Anomalous Phenomena)
56 Telemann Square
Kidbrook
London SE3

Fortean Times
96 Mansfield Road
London NW3 2HX

Society for Psychical Research
1 Adam & Eve Mews
London W8 6UG